ENERGETIC HEALING

Embracing the Life Force

ARNIE LADE

LOTUS

COPYRIGHT 1998 By ARNIE LADE

Cover art and design: Carola Höchst-Teague
Photography: David Connell
Design & Page Layout: Carola Höchst-Teague

First Edition, 1998

Printed in the United States of America

Library of Congress Cataloging-in-Publication-Data
Lade, Arnie

includes bibliographical references.
ISBN 0-914955-46-2   98-67863
                                                 CIP

Published by:
Lotus Press, P.O. Box 325, Twin Lakes, Wisconsin 53181

Table of Contents

Acknowledgements

I wish to thank John Upledger, Alastair Pirie and Judy Trost for their gracious reviews of this book during its development. Thanks as well to Ken Bloomfield for his many insightful comments and suggestions; he is a true master of words. Special heartfelt thanks go to my wife, Diane, for her excellent artwork and skill at capturing images as they were intended. Lastly, I wish to honor my many patients and students who throughout the years have taught me so much about energy, life, love and healing.

Forword

Years ago, when people would ask me how I saw the future of the forest and its ancient Knowledge - I answered that I felt that there was very little hope about preserving this Knowledge. I felt the same way about all the ancient Knowledge disappearing around the world. I knew that this Knowledge which nature imparts to all things from its most intimate being was no longer being honored or understood by humanity. Feeling sad, I began to give up and withdraw from this lonely struggle. I decided to turn my back on the human world and just enjoy what was left. But during my time in the forest I received messages to continue what I then felt to be a loosing battle - to keep on trying to preserve this Knowledge and share it with those that would listen. I asked the forest for guidance - to find people who also see the priceless value of nature, as I do. Answers began to unfold and unique individuals like Arnie Lade crossed my path. Arnie has dedicated his life to learning and teaching. His diverse background incorporates the disciplines of Chinese, Ayurvedic and South American medicines. His day to day experiences with patients has made him a respected healer and a knowledgeable teacher.

After a lifetime of studying Peruvian "traditional" medicine, I can gratefully say that Arnie's pioneering work is continually breaking important ground for the rest of us in the field of natural medicine. Arnie takes us on a journey of inner exploration that allows us to reclaim an intimate wisdom of ourselves. It is my pleasure to share his latest work with you.

Dr. Jose Gonzalo Cabanillas
Isula Biological Preserve
Amazon River
Iquitos, Peru

Introduction

"Seeking not to follow the footsteps of the ancient ones, I seek that which they attained." - Basho

This book is about something that was almost lost, something that humanity could not measure, explain or appreciate. Gradually people no longer talked about it, and in time was almost forgotten. Some traditional cultures still referred to it, but most of us did not give these old ideas serious thought; we had our own concerns and explanations. This is how it was until we started to run out of answers; only then did we look around and see the emptiness resulting from the loss of all that we once had.

For most of us, the world of today is quite different from that of our ancestors. Humanity's effort to understand and shape the world around us has literally transformed life on earth, not only for ourselves but for all species. Today, the oceans, skies, and continents have all been explored; nature has been mastered as never before, and the planets and moon are now within our reach. We have more collective wealth than ever before and supposedly more leisure time to enjoy it.

At the same time, we appear to be desperately searching for a pathway out of the looming crisis in the environment, the social pathology of our cities, and the ever new and virulent diseases that afflict us. We live in a global culture that is troubled by a host of disquieting problems: economic disparity, drugs, crime, racial and religious tensions, and the list goes on.

This century has not been an easy one. We have suffered two world wars and countless others, subjected ourselves to scientific revolution and social turmoil, and survived the collapse and struggle to regain order (from feudalism to fascism, to communism and democracy.) We have also abandoned in large numbers the religions we once followed, and endured an endless stream of change that is largely driven by materialistic sentiments.

You can argue that we have gained so much, but I lament all that has been lost. What untold wisdom, culture, and habitats have we abandoned? What fellow creatures amongst the animals, birds, fish and plants have we forsaken and removed from the surface of this delicate planet we call earth?

Perhaps our quest for knowledge and dominion over nature has improved the quality of life for some, but it has not given life more meaning. We have alienated ourselves from one another, replaced spirituality with materialism and wonder with reason. Most of us are no longer content with nature; we have become strangers in our own home.

Yet, the horizon is not all dark and foreboding. There are still many people in search of meaning and purpose who wish to pursue a life of harmony within themselves, with each other and nature. I see many positive developments, such as the emergence of a concern for the environment, the reawakening of spirituality based upon respect for all paths, and the renewed interest in healing practices which embrace our innate wholeness, including the mind and emotions. In my opinion, these three - ecology, spirituality and healing - are, today, the main currents of a New Renaissance, one that is global in nature.

I also find heartening the recent development in science of holistic models which enable us to transcend the reductionist and mechanistic thinking of earlier science. For too long science has looked down the microscope to study the building blocks of nature. The drive to discover the workings of nature and harness her forces led scientists to the heart of matter, only to find that matter itself arises from and is shaped by energy. A leading principle in this new science, quantum theory, imagines the raw material of the universe to be flows of energy occurring within a unified field in which matter is only one manifestation.

Certainly humanity has benefited from science in terms of technology; yet there is a feeling of detachment and cold materialism inherent in the scientific approach. In the old scientific paradigm, analysis, logic, and rational and critical thinking are believed to yield the greatest rewards in the acquisition of knowledge. Meanwhile perception, non-linear, holistic and intuitive thinking are given short change. In the pursuit of information, one could find oneself discovering "more and more about less and less." Knowledge, as the functional relationship of processes, challenges a greater insight. Only recently have some pioneers in scientific thought been able to turn the microscope around. Instead of a narrow focus on matter, a broadening of vision about life and the cohesion of phenomena has emerged, a vision that is based upon perception that embraces both thought and feeling.

In particular, I draw hope from the growing acceptance of the Gaia hypothesis. This theory brings together proof that the dense network of organic and inorganic portions of the Earth's surface form a single system, a kind of mega-organism. From this perspective, ours is a living planet, Gaia - the ancient goddess who is recognizable as an archetype of the Earth Mother in perhaps all religions - in which human beings are a part of a whole. Our destiny as human beings lies not only in what we do for ourselves but is interdependent with all of Gaia.

A similar shift is occurring in the healing arts. Modern biomedicine has left many people feeling alienated and distrustful, for the intrinsic flaws of the current medical approach are starting to become increasingly visible. The search for a cure for every identifiable disease-causing pathogen - be it the virus that causes AIDS or the common cold, or some renegade cancer gene, or a noxious poison or bacteria - is seemingly more and more elusive. Modern medicine is unable to keep up with this kind of "search and destroy" strategy. There are simply not enough magic bullets being produced for all the conceivable pathogens that can harm the physical body. For each successful cure there exists new and unsolved diseases which require a search for an elusive pathogen. Furthermore, living pathogens are themselves unstable; they undergo mutation and change, becoming resistant to the drugs that were once effective against them. Modern medicine is like a law enforcement agency that is unable to cope with an ever increasing number of new and repeat offenders. The simple enforcement of laws does not by itself solve the problem of crime.

Do not get me wrong. The material search for curing disease is an important and noble task. Unfortunately, this task is currently over emphasized in health care. The causes of disease are not to be found in matter alone, for illness often arises from the mind and spirit of a human being. To truly understand health and illness, medicine must look beyond physical causative agents and embrace the wholeness of human life. Medicine cannot go on pretending that it is fixing a machine. Instead, a thinking and feeling person who is living in his or her unique environment may need a more comprehensive system of treatment.

The essential problem is that medicine is still locked into the old science. Diseases are still believed to originate from chemical, biological, genetic or physical factors. That which permeates, shapes and guides matter is disregarded. Energy, I believe, is the missing factor.

Throughout life, from conception to death, the physical body is held together by a life force or energy which has a patterning influence. When this force finally withdraws, death occurs, leaving the body unable to maintain its form. The matter within the lifeless body decomposes, returning to the elemental forms from which it arose. We need to consider a hidden essence with causal character-istics as its expression.

This life force or energy shapes our bodies and creates their structure; it heals our wounds and allows body, mind, and spirit to function as a unit. In earlier times the sum of this energy was called the life body, or etheric body. I call it the energetic terrain. All living beings - plants, animals and humans - have an energy or life force working within them.

How could we ever understand human life or any other form of life by simply studying its material components? The beauty, meaning and wonder of life can only be found by perceiving the whole. Life is about an unseen inner world as much as it is about the visible forms they embody. Life exists within a relationship of many parts to the whole and the whole to the many parts.

In my opinion, the modern schism between what psy-chology calls mind and emotions, and what medicine calls anatomy and physiology, and what religion calls spirit or soul - is based on the fact that the life force is no longer considered an integral part of the human constitution. I have no doubt that energy is the unifying factor between mind, body and spirit. This book is a study on the role and patterning of energy within human life.

In my own life, I have pursued a study of the energetic terrain for more than 25 years. I have studied various western and eastern healing arts, from polarity therapy to acupuncture, disciplines that still embrace the concept of energy or life force. I have also been blessed with the opportunity to study with various spiritual teachers and traditions, thereby gaining new perspectives on the inner realm. Yet, I can honestly say that the more I have experienced and learned, the more I realize the vastness of the subject and the difficulty of describing its terrain.

The underlying philosophy of this work is firmly rooted in the ancient teachings of Asia, notably Taoism, Yoga and Tantra, as well as their complementary healing arts: Chinese medicine and Ayurveda. These traditions still honor the role of energy in the human constitution. I have also drawn upon important elements within the modern disciplines of science, biomedicine, osteopathy and psychology to describe or interpret certain observations about energy. I believe no single way of viewing the world guarantees the solution to its mysteries. Each vantage point offers a truth of its own, and together the essential, though varied, aspects of knowledge can shed a new and better light upon this important topic.

Throughout the text, I have consciously followed an integrative and eclectic approach, one that is clear, orderly and relatively free of culturally specific ideas. I have tried to illuminate the ancient jewels of truth by reinterpreting and bringing them into the language, knowledge and images of the present. In other places, I have correlated modern knowledge and insights with ancient truths. In this way I hope a more complete image of the energetic terrain emerges.

In this book, I intend to map out the inner landscape and to explain how this subtle energy manifests in varying forms and functions. I will explain the role of energy in uniting the mind, body and spirit, as well as how this new energy concept can be used in healing. Also, at the end of each chapter, a simple yet powerful exercise is described for the benefit of the reader who wishes to experience and begin to work with this inner energy.

I trust this book will shed new light upon the energetic terrain. I believe this new model of energy is an important bridge in transforming our current understanding of human existence and healing. My hope is that it will act as a stimulus for your own inner discovery of energy. In the end, may this work contribute to humanity's emerging renaissance!

CHAPTER ONE

The Sacred Terrain

"Whatever the inward darkness may have been to which the shamans descended in their trances, the same must lie within ourselves, nightly visited in our sleep." - Joseph Campbell

My inner life shapes how I perceive the world around me, while the outer world continually influences, forms and confirms my being. The outer and inner are parts of a whole: that which can be found in one will be found in the other. This is a truth that I have come to know and respect with greater appreciation.

We know, for example, that human beings from the earliest times have sensed that certain locations are sacred. At these sites human beings intuitively feel the presence and convergence of powerful forces, and thus we sanctify these places out of respect for their virtuous ambience. In those places a church, temple or mosque has often been built, embellished with sacred paintings, designs or other religious works of art. In more primitive cultures, natural formations like caves were revered and adorned with drawings rich in meaning. In the Americas, the indigenous people constructed circles made of stones (medicine wheels) to attest to a site's sacredness, or in some cases special sites have deities or guardian spirits attributed to them.

1-1 Medicine Wheel

Sacred to Native Americans, medicine wheels are found throughout the Americas in locations of special significance or power. The wheel depicted is based upon the one found in the Big Horn Mountains in Wyoming, USA. Over 35 meters in diameter the wheel contains 28 spokes radiating from a central cairn with 6 smaller cairns around the periphery. These landmarks orientate the wheel to the key directions and astrological events. Circles reflect the essential movements of life, just as sun, moon, stars and seasons reveal the essential movements of the cosmos.

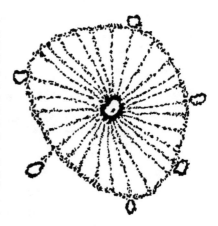

At these sites of consecrated and concentrated power, the inner life of an individual can emerge because a psychological separation from life's ordinary outer events occurs. Our connection to the realm of spirit is thereby renewed. In many ways these sites function like spiritual wombs to nurture the essence within a person. Sacred sites also offer the community a social forum for worshiping together, for sharing religious teachings and for healing.

Personally, I too have felt a special affinity for certain places. In those places, a closeness and clarity is felt with the beauty, harmony and mysteries of life. For me, such places have often been in nature, particularly in the mountains. Other places also come to mind: the long-forgotten Taoist temple ruin which I once found on a pilgrimage in China, or a modern-day pyramid-like church in Brasilia that I recently visited. On occasion, I yearn to return to one of these sites, to renew and gather together my inner life. We all have our own special places.

Just as we can experience an external spiritual reality, a sacred terrain also exists within human existence, a terrain that is composed of spirit, mind, energy and form. In this chapter, some common themes will be discussed, including how energy has been understood and described in traditional cultures. I hope to show that humanity has a rich heritage regarding energy which we can draw upon. Ideas from this heritage will be more closely examined and re-framed throughout the book.

Throughout history, many divergent societies have developed teachings that describe and chart this inner terrain, a realm that is largely experiential in nature. For each culture the portrayal of the inner realm is described according to its own paradigm or world view. Each paradigm is composed of all the spiritual, mythological, social and healing beliefs of that culture or group, as well as the language through which they are expressed.

Unfortunately these teachings become obscured by a symbolism that is only understandable to the initiate of that particular teaching. This problem is compounded by the fact that our era has witnessed the rapid loss of traditional knowledge due to the advance of our modern global civilization. Every day the traditional way of life of indigenous people (as found in the remote corners of this earth's rain-forests, arctic snows and distant highlands) is being destroyed by new diseases, unmitigated consumer-materialism, and alien religions, as well as concepts that are being propagated by the dominant cultures of our time.

I believe the primitive mythological and archaic interpretations of reality represent an important intuitive and feeling capacity in humanity's understanding of life. In stark contrast to most traditional knowledge is the modern use of scientific hypotheses and thought-models of reality which are generally devoid of feeling. For example, the current computer revolution and interest in space is more cerebral then visceral, more thinking then feeling in nature. Of course, the intuitive and feeling modes of awareness are and always will be recoverable within the human experience and to a large extent this mode has been embraced by the artists, writers and healers in modern society.

Most traditions describe the existence of a life force or energy at the heart of the inner terrain. This energy has been given many names: lung (Tibetans), ka (Egyptians), prana (Hindu), baraka (Sufis), mingo (Africans), mana (Polynesians), qi (Chinese), ki (Japanese), pneuma (classical Greek), lil (Mayans) and so on. Usually much importance and respect is given to the energy within. Energy is seen as a sacred force, for without it body and mind would be unable to exist, and the spirit would be unable to manifest within the human form. More explicit information will be given on this subject in the next chapter.

Asian Traditions

One of the world's great teachings in terms of the inner sacred and energetic terrain is Taoism, which arose in China more than 2,500 years ago. Taoism is a philosophical and spiritual movement that has greatly influenced Chinese culture. The fine arts, literature, medicine, sciences and martial arts of China continue to owe their soul to Taoism. Taoism offers a unique vision of the human being's energetic constitution, a vision that is derived from an intensive study of humanity and nature. In relationship to the themes addressed in this work, two Taoist concepts are noteworthy. These are the idea of a primal duality that exists within all things, referred to as the Yin-Yang philosophy, and the belief that each person has a subtle energy called Qi (pronounced "chee" like in the word cheese) which circulates within the body.

Other wellsprings of knowledge that I have drawn upon for inspiration are the two Asian traditions of Tantra and Yoga. These traditions are native to India, with roots firmly planted in the Hindu and Buddhist religions. Furthermore, the medical tradition of India, Ayurveda, incorporates and complements the essential ideas of Yoga and Tantra. Basic to the teachings of Yoga and Tantra is the notion that within each person there exists a subtle, formative sphere or body, invisible to ordinary sense perception. This subtle sphere is intimately linked with consciousness and is organized around a system known as the sushumna and chakras in the Sanskrit language. Essentially the sushumna is viewed as the inner divine core in human beings, extremely subtle and immaterial in nature. Along the core there are seven chakras or psychic centers that differentiate consciousness. Indeed, the Indian model offers a compelling description of humanity's deepest layer within the inner terrain, one that connects with other similar structural insights.

In Appendices I and II an outline is given, respectively, of the Chinese and Indian spiritual and healing traditions that relate to this book's theme. I encourage those readers unfamiliar with these Asian traditions to read these two Appendices first, after completing this chapter.

Traditions in the Americas

The famous American mythologist Joseph Campbell has written extensively , in his many books, on the inner sacred and energetic landscape from a cross-cultural and mythological perspective. According to Campbell, India's sushumna-chakra system metaphorically represents the unfolding of human consciousness and the body's vital energy through marked stages.

In essence, Campbell perceives that this inner dimension incorporates energetic and somatic pathways, human biological drives, aspects of time, psychological states, spiritual and mystic realms and the relationship of humanity to nature, all within a journey towards wholeness. The word "wholeness" implies a state of incompleteness which arouses a desire for integration at some level yet to be discovered.

However, even more fascinating is the fact that Campbell utilizes the Indian sushumna-chakra model as a foundation for exploring parallel concepts and archetypal images within the various ancient Eurasian civilizations of Assyria, Sumer, China, Tibet, and so forth, as well as the Aztec and Navaho cultures in the Americas. He was particularly impressed by the similarities between the Indian description and that of the American native culture of the Navahos. This particular North American tribe utilized sand paintings as a vehicle to describe an individual's spiritual and healing journey along what they termed the mystical Pollen Path. This whole procedure is strikingly similar to East Indian and Tibetan sand paintings in both intention and practice. In his book, *The Inner Reaches of Outer Space: Metaphors as Myth and as Religion*, Campbell makes the following comment:

"One can only wonder, considering, as I have been considering for some forty-odd years, the likeness, both in breadth and in depth, of the two constellations of metaphorical images of the Old World and the New, whether the human psyche can possibly be so thoroughly programmed that these two all but identical constellations might indeed have arisen independently in the separated hemispheres of our planet. Some idea of the astonishing intimacy in detail of the great convergence (if that, indeed, is what it is) may be gained simply by confronting, as though of one and the same mystical heritage, such an example of New World iconography as the Navaho sand painting and the wisdom-lore of India's Old World yoga."

An indigenous Mayan from Mexico named Hunbatz Men, an eminent authority on his culture, states in his book *Secrets of Mayan Science/Religion* that the Mayan culture also developed a broad vision of the inner dimension. For the Mayans the chaclas (strangely similar both in meaning and phonetics with the Sanskrit word chakra) are the foundation of the human spiritual and energetic terrain. According to Hunbatz Men the word chacla also refers, on a macrocosmic level, to the force that moves and forms the Milky Way. To the Mayans there is also a seven-fold differentiation of the chaclas within the subtle sphere's core.

Various indigenous cultures in the Americas, including Mayan, Inca, and Cherokee, believe that humankind had galactic origins. Specifically the seeds of the human consciousness, as we know it, came from the Pleiades, the star cluster with seven visible stars. Traditionally, it has been told that these ancestors from space intermixed with the highest, but definitely animal-like, primates on earth. Human beings, as we are today, are the result of this marriage. Indeed the great cities and temples of the Mayan, Aztec and Incan culture all aligned their orientation perfectly to the Pleiades they worshiped. To these people the manifold aspects and powers of the spirit and psyche resonate in a differentiated system of seven, symbolic of the celestial origins of human consciousness. Thus the outer and inner sacred terrain form mirror images - the seven inner chaclas and the outer seven stars of the Pleiades.

Interestingly, in both India and China the Pleiades also occupy an important position. Both of these civilizations use a system of astrology that includes twenty-eight lunar mansions, roughly comprised of the same groupings of stars. The starting point of celestial reckoning of time, in both traditions, began with the appearance of the constellation centered on the Pleiades during the vernal equinox, somewhere between 1500 and 2000 B.C.

How can we explain the emergence of common ideas and practices in geographically separated cultures? Usually, two main explanations are put forward, one historical and the other psychological. In some cases both explanations may apply.

The historical argument suggests that information, technology and customs are passed on from one culture or society to another through direct contact, frequently through trade and/or conquest. For example, gunpowder was originated in China from where it went slowly to Europe and then to the Americas after Columbus.

In the same way many civilizations propagated their own spiritual, medical and healing teachings to the cultures they came in contact with. Sometimes adoption of new ideas, words and practices was rapid and at other times evolved slowly over many generations. For example, the Hinduization of the Malay peninsula, Indochina and the islands of present day western Indonesia occurred around 100 A.D. when Hindu culture, economics, philosophy, and its diverse spiritual and healing practices influenced the cultures it encountered. Later, the Muslims came with their unique world view and practices, often completely altering the previous way of life.

Many years ago I was in Bali, a tiny island in Indonesia that is the last remnant of the once powerful Hindu culture in South-East Asia. The Muslim invasion came to its shore but could not conquer this island. Bali has an interesting blend of a Hindu culture that has been cut off from other Hindu lands for hundreds of years, combined with its indigenous beliefs and practices that may go back thousands of years. I have seen ancient Vedic rituals in

Bali that perhaps no longer exist in India, the home of Hinduism itself.

Of course, controversy does arise from age to age as to which culture originated this or that particular teaching. Unfortunately, most civilizations have tended to see themselves as the original or chosen people and in turn exhibit an ethnocentric world view, claiming to be the source of wisdom and refinement of culture. For example, history has shown that the British, Chinese, Greek, Mayans and East Indians, among others, have all held notions about their civilization's uniqueness.

Then there is the psychological interpretation that these culturally distinct traditions and teachings arose from individuals within the society who somehow communed with humanity's transpersonal infraconscious, a hidden wellspring of awareness and knowledge inside us all. Dr. Carl Jung, an early pioneer in modern psychology, calls this the transpersonal or collective unconscious. I prefer to use the word infraconscious instead of unconscious because infra, meaning below, refers to consciousness at a different level, not its absence. These awakenings into the transpersonal infraconscious appear to occur approximately within the same time period in various places on the planet, thus providing a psychological explanation why two societies isolated by their geography can have remarkably parallel myths, spiritual beliefs, practices of medicine, discoveries in technology and so on.

The Global Use of Acupuncture

This idea of collective similarities in human life and society is revealed in the repetition of certain medical practices and concepts throughout the globe. Acupuncture, for example, is generally considered to be a healing art of Chinese origin, yet I have found this practice to exist in South America among indigenous tribes in an archaic form. These native people (such as the Mapuches of southern Chile and certain Amazonian tribes), living in simple conditions, utilized the sharp thorns of trees and bushes to pierce specific points to treat all sorts of ailments. This technique is apparently passed down through oral teachings. In fact, there is physical evidence of acupuncture being used in South America in the ancient past, well before the Incas. In Dr. Javier Cabrera Darquea's book *The Message of the Engraved Stones of Ica* there are photographs of scenes etched on stones of various sizes that were found in Peru. These rocks clearly show ancient people using acupuncture for healing and surgery.

Likewise, according to numerous reports there existed in Sri Lanka and south India a system of acupuncture that predated the arrival of the first Chinese trading missions. The Ola manuscript reported to be from around 200 B.C. states, "Be mindful what the pulse reveals before thou dost apply, the needle science of Iswara revealed in days gone by." Today there can still be found in Sri Lanka

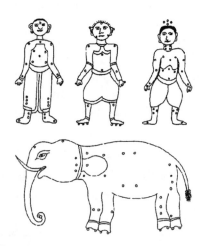

1-2 Sri Lankan Acupuncture

The above figures drawn from classical Sri Lankan texts show the location of important *nila* or acupuncture points on both human beings and elephants.

and south India practitioners of this indigenous form of acupuncture.

The principal difference between the various forms of acupuncture found throughout the world and the Chinese variety is that the ancient Chinese advanced a concept of energy flows or meridians. Essentially, the Chinese envisioned that the various points on the body (that could be pierced by fine needles, heated or massaged) were strategic locations along meridians where its energy or Qi was accessible. This network of meridians not only circulates near the skin's surface but also communicates with the internal organs and structures. The acupuncture points acted as portals through which the body and mind could be harmonized. In comparison, the non-Chinese forms of acupuncture do not appear to have evolved such an all embracing energetic concept around the practice of acupuncture.

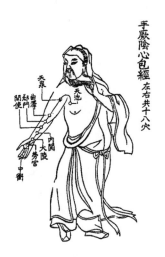

1-3 Classical Acupuncture Meridian

This clasical drawing depicts the external route of the Heart Protector meridian and its nine points. In total the human body possess twelve bilateral and two unilateral meridians which circulate Qi along their routes.

Although the healing art of acupuncture seems to be unique in each of the three above-mentioned cultures (China, South Asia and South America), it is possible that this technique appeared in all three places during the same epoch. I do not believe a historical explanation makes sense as to why acupuncture is found in these diverse lands and cultures; rather the answer may be found within the transpersonal infraconscious. Nevertheless, it was in the Chinese civilization that acupuncture developed roots to flower eventually as a complex and important healing art. Perhaps China's literary tradition in medicine had a lot to do with Chinese acupuncture's exceptional development throughout Asia and, more recently, the entire world.

In this age of communication, where the planet is increasingly like a global village, we are just beginning to discover humanity's collective similarities as a species. In this chapter I have tried to show how the inner sacred and energetic terrain, which embraces the whole self, is viewed and utilized throughout the world in surprisingly similar ways. Keeping all of this in mind, I would like to explore in Chapter Two the enigma of birth, death and rebirth before looking at the energetic terrain proper.

Now, as a method of realizing some of the insights I have described in Chapter One, try the exercise called Finding the Sacred Abode described on the next page.

Exercise 1
Finding the Sacred Abode

Visualization is a form of guided imagery that can be used to expand our awareness and to recover lost memories. After each chapter, I will describe an exercise that ties into a theme from that chapter. The exercises will embrace different aspects of the energetic terrain. A few, like this exercise, will be related more to spirit and consciousness; later exercises will focus directly on specific energetic systems. All of them are designed to increase awareness of the subtle dimension that exists within us all. You may wish to pre-record an exercise on a machine and play it back to yourself while you are in the prescribed position. If you do this, please leave time on the recording for contemplation and your imagery to emerge.

This particular exercise explores the place within us all that can be used as a refuge, a peaceful inner temple, where we are safe, contented and alone. We all require such a place to withdraw into, from time to time, so that we can live life fully, with independence and inner strength.

Begin by finding a nice comfortable and quiet place in which you can sit or lie down. This exercise will take about 20 minutes. Rest with your arms and legs uncrossed so that your energy flows remain unimpeded. Close your eyes and commence by noticing any physical sensations arising from your body. Just acknowledge these impressions and let them recede into the background of your awareness. Follow this by checking the flow of your thoughts; again just accept and suspend any preoccupations for now. Do the same with your feelings. Slowly let sensations, feelings and thoughts all recede into the background.

Now, start to look around in your body for a door to an inner space that is safe, secure, and intimate. Ask the door to open; go inside. There you will find a special box or album full of memories, feelings and images of special moments, people, events, and places that have given your life meaning. Open this album and let your mind and spirit recall those experiences; simply let what comes into your awareness be there. Perhaps there will be just one memory or

21

many; trust whatever emerges from within yourself to be what is needed. Sense any change in your awareness or feelings that may manifest. Then in a few moments ask yourself these questions:

Do I feel any change?
What quality is emerging?
Is there a loving presence or sense of power manifest?
Where does this inner space reside in my physical body?

Now ask yourself: Is there a wish or hope that I can put into this sacred space? Something that I would like to cultivate and let grow in the depth of my being? If so, silently imprint it into your album. Slowly close the box or album and then gently turn away and gracefully leave this inner space. Remember to close the door behind you as you leave. Allow your breath to deepen and let any new found inner awareness or quality to be dispersed throughout your whole body.

Slowly open your eyes. Notice how you are feeling. Give time to integrate your experience for a while. Try to recall this place whenever you need inner strength, support or love.

CHAPTER TWO

Birth, Death and Rebirth

"You are what you think, having become what you thought." - Buddha

There is a human tendency to want a plan which will lay life's journey out for us. Most of us want to know and have a sense of certainty about what may lie ahead. Our doubts and anxieties may even provoke the need to have someone or something show us the way, be it a teacher, priest, guru or sacred text. Granted, we do at times need guidance and reassurance along the road of life, but the great mysteries - about life and death, God and human purpose - can never be totally explained or conveyed. They are a matter of inner realization and perception.

The difficult truth is that we are or seem to be solitary. All of one's thoughts, emotions, dreams, fears and sufferings can never be fully shared. I know that I create my own reality within each moment of my life. This is both my freedom and bondage.

Throughout the rest of this book, I will try to explain to you what I have understood about the energetic terrain, using words, images and illustrations as my medium. I will speak in general terms, sharing with you what I know, what I have experienced, and what I have not yet understood. Please take in the information as you would a painting or story.

Remember, these are my experiences and understanding; do not accept them as being true unless or until you can confirm them through your own experience. I am not trying to create an image for you to believe in or subscribe to. Rather I hope my descriptions will be a guide along your own inner journey of discovery. Perhaps your experience will be different; this is perfectly natural. Although we all possess similar energetic features, each person possesses his or her own unique configuration of energy. Your energetic terrain is as original as your thoughts, feelings, physical form and gestures. I will be describing the energetic terrain from this perspective. I believe it is good to belong to a whole while maintaining individuality.

Let us start our exploration of energy by looking at the beginning and ending of human life. How did we get here and where do we go when we die? Answering these questions and others will give us a clue to how energy manifests throughout life.

Beyond This Life

I have always felt that I am no stranger to this earth. Many times, I have experienced a familiarity in certain places or with particular people or in specific situations. There has been a powerful feeling of deja vu, even though I had never been there, known them, or experienced it before. All my life, I have felt certain that this life is not my only life, that death cannot be the end. I have at times remembered things that could not be related to this life, but must be memories of past times and lives. I felt great comfort when I found that other people and societies also shared this belief.

In a way, birth and death are reflections of each other. I have seen both in this life. I know we are affected by our own births, sometimes emotionally even scared by them. Does the quality of our lives determine our death? I believe it does. Birth and death are potentially profound and healing experiences; they are transitions into and out of this reality.

Once, a few years back, my father was hospitalized for a severe bout of fluid retention in relation to an ongoing heart condition. On my first visit to see him, I had an unforgettable experience. As I entered the room I noticed two other gentlemen sharing his room. One of them was obviously quite old, apparently in his 90's, and the other a little younger, perhaps in his 70's. Anyway, I sat down and started to chat with my dad. It was hard for him to talk too much, so I carried the conversation along. After about 15 minutes in the room I began to have an odd sensation. I felt something important was going on behind me! Turning around, I saw the old man fidgeting with his oxygen tube and withdrawing it from his nose. Then he slowly lowered his head and rested it on his pillow. He looked peaceful with his face relaxed and mouth open. That is not unusual, I thought.

I resumed my conversation with my father, yet my awareness continued to be drawn to this old man. All of a sudden, I don't know how, but I began to perceive that he was leaving his body right then and there! I sensed that he had stopped breathing. I closed my eyes and in my inner vision I saw a blue orb of light leaving and floating out over his body on the hospital bed. I mentioned this to my dad. He looked over and said nothing, perhaps not knowing whether to believe me. I asked him about the old man. He said that he was an old sailor and that his wife and son had only left the room an hour before I came in. I decided not to interfere or say anything. Let him have a peaceful death; no one else can do anything about it now, I thought to myself.

As I sat with my father I internally sensed, conversed with and prayed for the old man's spirit in the room.

Finally, after more than a half hour I decided to go over to his body and check the pulse. Before I could touch his hand the third person in the room spoke to me in an agitated manner and told me that I shouldn't bother the old man. Couldn't I see that he was sleeping? Okay, I replied, I'll leave him alone. I sat back down by my father's side, and chatted some more. When I no longer felt the presence of the old man's spirit, I decided that I could go. Before I left, I told my dad to tell the nurse about the old man when she comes in. The next day my father said the nurse came in 10 minutes later and pronounced the man dead. My father remembered this event and would talk to me about it from time to time. He was impressed by the peacefulness of the old man's death. This experience seemed to give my father strength in his own journey towards death.

What the Ancients Tell Us

In many cultures the soul or spirit is thought to choose, through intention or attraction, its particular parents. One such culture is the Tibetan. Indeed, the famous text *The Tibetan Book of the Dead* (Bardo Thodol), written in the fourteenth century, instructs an aspirant to master the transitions of death and rebirth in order to achieve the most appropriate situation and body for spiritual growth in the next life.

The Tibetan Book of the Dead states that the disincarnate consciousness or spirit, due to karma (i.e. cause and effect, see below), gravitates through conscious intention or unconscious attraction towards the energies generated in the sexual union of its future parents. When the physical connection actualizes itself into a fertilized egg, a slow bonding happens between the disincarnate consciousness (or soul, as others would say) and its future body. This bonding is completed either prior to or during the birth process, depending on the spiritual evolution of the new-born being. But even then, full awareness is obscured in the dreamlike state experienced by the infant and young child.

In Asia, most traditional societies acknowledge the existence of pivotal points in nature which usually occur in cycles, like the changes of seasons and phases of the moon. This is why much sanctity is given to the major celestial transitions, in the form of the lunar and seasonal rituals. Traditional societies also honor pivotal points in human life with rites of passage in birth, puberty, marriage, old age and death. In those spiritual traditions such moments hold extreme import and mystery, and are opportunities for influencing deeper levels of human existence. Also, profound dreams or meditative experiences, as well as powerful life events such as seeing one's child being born or a near-death experience, may have such personal import as to radically change one's personality. Thus, through such events we can be reborn, not through the spirit into a new form, but through the psyche into a new awareness and outlook.

Sogyal Rimpoche, a renowned Tibetan Buddhist teacher and author of *The Tibetan Book of Living and Dying,* says that these pivotal points, called bardos in Tibetan, are potent opportunities for spiritual awakening. Indeed the whole of existence is considered to go through four great bardos of interlinked realities: life, dying and death, the time after death and rebirth.

Of course, the Buddhist and Hindu traditions of Asia are not the only cultures that accept rebirth as a reality, for this concept has been embraced by many people and cultures throughout the ages, such as Hasidic Jews, certain Native American tribes like the Cherokee, and Taoists, to name a few. Yet Tibetan Buddhism offers us a richly detailed guide for the journey through the great bardo of death. It is a living guide that has been researched by innumerable sages and masters who have made the journey and described the landscape.

Rebirth

I should note that Buddhists do not believe in the reincarnation of a soul as an immortal, independent or unchanging entity that passes from one life to the next. Rather, Buddhists maintain that consciousness, or mind, exists as an evolving continuum that is reborn in countless existences. According to the principle of cause and effect, they believe the subtle changes that occur within consciousness are a direct result of its interaction with reality (all phenomena within this world and the universe surrounding us). Furthermore, when the physical body dies, only the most subtle aspects of consciousness are thought to be carried forward into the next existence.

I do not really know if a pure spirit exists that is identical within us all, or if there is an evolving consciousness that is different with each incarnation. This is beyond my present understanding. I would argue, however, that the concept of soul need not be static, and that it could embrace the Buddhist notion of mind. Throughout this text I have used the words spirit, soul and consciousness interchangeably, giving them this liberal interpretation.

Also, I have problems accepting the concept of rebirth of human beings into or out of the animal kingdom, which the Buddhists and Hindus advocate. In my view, the human, animal, plant, and mineral kingdoms all manifest within their own field, within which a particular form remains for all rebirths or transformations. Thus, I believe human consciousness remains, while on earth, bound to the human domain. I believe in the orderliness of the appropriate divisions, or "realms."

Four Kingdoms

When we think about the four kingdoms (mineral, plant, animal and human), it is quite natural to see the difference between human beings and the processes inherent in mineral and plant kingdoms, but we have more problems differentiating ourselves from the animal realm.

The mineral kingdom does not have life as we recognize it, but it does have subtle forces that work through it. Over long periods of time they create change, a rather slow metamorphosis within the earth herself. Plants, on the other hand, are filled with abundant life force. In a plant's seed is hidden the whole of the plant, out of which some inner force brings forth the leaf, stem, roots, flower and fruit all in good order. In the animal realm the metamorphic stages of life begin with the sperm and egg. In the plant, the seed and flower are in natural polarity to each other, while in the animal the egg and the new egg cells produced by the adult form a polarity. Yet, there is more in this animal life than what appears in the plant. There is an awareness of being that is intimately connected to its environment and governed by instinctual knowledge and desire. Certainly, an animal feels, senses and thinks, and perhaps because of this we human beings often find kinship with them.

Science would have us believe that human beings have evolved from animals and that at best we are really only higher animals. I do not believe this to be entirely true. In my view, humanity stands apart from animals. A plant lives and can sense its environment. The animal, in addition to living and sensing, has feelings and desires; but the human being carries something that makes him or her capable of self knowledge. The ideas of responsibility, freedom, creative expression, compassion, and morality are evidence of a different journey humanity must walk upon.

I do not want to venture too far from the theme of this book, but I would like to add that I consider that the four kingdoms - mineral, plant, animal and human - form uninterrupted evolutionary stages through which the divine creative force manifests respectively the body, life, feeling, and spirit qualities on earth. Human beings embody all four qualities. We are not set completely apart from the other kingdoms. We are a divine creative expression that gives this earth meaning and wholeness.

Conception

Returning to the theme of human biological conception, the first moments witness the fusion of egg and sperm physically. While there is an amazing physical process going on, there are also subtle forces operating within this process. Chinese classical philosophy and medicine portray this biological fusion as a union of two things: the parent's Qi and essence (jing). The term essence refers to the biological matrix within the visible sperm and egg that determines the inherited body type, including metabolism, basal vitality, DNA, and other physical qualities. In contrast, Qi - in this case specifically called original Qi (yuan qi) - refers to the unique life force within the individual's ancestral lineage and human species in general. Original Qi also transmits certain collective characteristics of psychological import, such as the instinctual knowledge necessary for survival and some aspects of our emotional makeup.

The result of this fusion is a unique physical form made up of genetic, biological and instinctual components. The disincarnate soul, which carries its own karmic patterning, will eventually animate and give true life to the material form of the evolving fetus. Thus the resulting personality and physical constitution are effectively the outcome of this mutual impression of matter, in the form of essence and Qi, and the spirit or soul.

Karma

At this point it may be appropriate to understand something about karma. Karma, put simply, is a chain of cause and effect. By itself, karma is neither "good" nor "bad," although we have a tendency to give this interpretation to it. Cosmically, all of creation operates by the principles of cause and effect. Ultimately there are no random events. Only our own inability to perceive the ordering of reality obscures this concept. As Albert Einstein once said: "God does not play dice with man." The universe operates according to the law of karma, an integrated design.

On the human level, karma is generated by the momentum of thought. Past tendencies and impressions produce the present thought patterns and personal reality. What is thought and done now creates the basis for one's future thoughts and reality. Furthermore, thoughts (and by extension, emotions and attitudes) are usually identified with the "self". In reality this is an illusionary self-image because thoughts themselves are being perceived by a seer, the pure undifferentiated spirit. Karma also occurs synchronistically, linking all creation together, and thus your thoughts affect your reality and vice versa. Karma is the root of all action, whether performed with intention or not. Karma literally means action. It is inherent in both "cause" and "effect."

The chain of events linking thought to karma is illustrated through the following formula: sow a thought, reap a desire; sow a desire, reap an action; sow an action, reap a habit; sow a habit, reap a character trait; sow a character trait, reap destiny; destiny is the fruit of karma.

One good example of a karmic pattern is that of cigarette smoking. A young person thinks about smoking after watching friends or advertisements on TV commercials. Thoughts arise, such as wouldn't it be cool to smoke, I'd really impress my friends, I wonder what it's like, and so on. This generates the desire to smoke, and repeated desire eventually results in the person trying it. Yet the desire and action to smoke returns, more and more often, in time becoming a habit, because satisfying the desire itself doesn't normally stop the flow of thought engendering the desire. This is because desire is the outcome of thought, not the reverse. Habits are tenacious in nature, eventually becoming part of the character. The smoker and others start to identify smoking with themselves. This in turn becomes their destiny to live out until another more appealing thought pattern emerges to change the flow of karma.

Usually, in time other emotions, attitudes and body signals become linked to the original thought projections. The awareness of most of these emotions, attitudes and body signals is repressed and removed from memory, remaining dormant within the personal infraconscious. In the case of smoking, feelings of guilt or rejection by non-smokers or the fear of cancer, or physically, a worrisome cough, may emerge. These new impressions add additional weight to the initial thoughts, creating complex patterns. But at each stage or moment it is the individual thoughts and the actions that follow that keep the momentum of karma going throughout life and beyond. Thus the sages say: if you want to know your past, look into your present condition; if you want to know your future, look at your present thoughts and desires.

Incarnating

During the process of incarnation, the spirit loses its awareness of past existences as it bonds with the new body. However, the memory of past lives and the disincarnate states of existence are not permanently forgotten; rather, they are stored in the causal sphere, including the deep recesses of the transpersonal infraconscious. In most individuals the memory of past lives and the non-embodied state will remain dormant throughout life. The young infant lives in a state of pure innocence without ego awareness. The "causal sphere" is a term used to denote the rarified aspect of consciousness or mind that survives death and is projected into a new body upon rebirth. Essentially, the causal sphere is the organized form of the spirit.

Altogether, a human being has four distinctive aspects or spheres (some authors have referred to them as bodies, but this term can be misleading). Besides the already mentioned causal sphere, there is the physical sphere made up of bodily matter that gives us our visible form. Then there is the not-so-visible energetic sphere or terrain wherein energy circulates, and finally the invisible mental sphere composed of the faculties: cognitive, rational, intuitive, and so on, as well as the ego and personal infraconscious.

The complete process of the spirit's identification or grounding within its new body normally occurs in stages. Initially the incarnate soul's memory becomes obscured quickly, followed by a slow and progressive re-emergence of awareness within its unfamiliar new physical form. This new awareness is co-dependent upon the actual inherited physical makeup of the body, as well as on psychological impressions derived from the mother and others. This whole process of re-emergence as a distinctive personality is more or less complete sometime between the fifth and seventh year after birth.

The Psychoenergetic Core

At the interface between the incarnating spirit and the developing physical form is an energetic potential, which I have termed the psychoenergetic core. In the east, the adept of Hindu or Buddhist Tantra would call this core the central conduit (sushumna), while a Taoist would call it the central vessel (zhong mai). The psychoenergetic core can be visualized as an energetic outline or space within the developing tissues of the physical body upon which the soul impresses itself, like a mold upon clay. Thus, the psychoenergetic core is intimately linked with the causal and mental spheres. Yet, it is also the hub and organizing force behind the whole of the energetic sphere.

The psychoenergetic core's primary purpose is to contain and orient the soul, as well as to embody and configure the karmic patterns and restrictions of one's previous and present lives. Essentially the core facilitates the soul's imprint upon and grounding into the physical body.

Along the core are seven differentiated centers, referred to in Tantra as the chakras. These centers are configurations of psychic forces and patterns, so that consciousness is organized, diffused, and concealed as certain karmic impressions are buried below the threshold of awareness. The psychoenergetic core, with its seven differentiated centers, is completely formed within the developing tissues of the embryo during the first few weeks. More will be said on this important energetic structure in the next two chapters.

The Stages of Dying and Death

In the east it is presumed that on the opposite end of life's journey, during the process of dying, the subtle energies from the physical body withdraw into the energetic terrain. Then the various energetic systems collapse into the psychoenergetic core from which they originally emerged. At the same time the mind starts to lose its cohesion, and only the refined aspects of consciousness are brought into the spirit which departs from the physical body upon death.

This whole process is metaphorically described in Indian and Tibetan philosophy as the separation and dissolution of the five great elements. The five elements (earth, water, fire, air and ether) embody all phenomena from the grossest to the most subtle. They are said to progressively lose their inherent cohesion and gradually merge together. First, the earth element becomes absorbed by the water element and the vision becomes blurred and the body heavy. Next the water element is absorbed by the fire element and the body cavities dry up; then the fire element is absorbed by the air element and the body loses heat. This is followed by the air element being absorbed into the ether element, which is accompanied by the cessation of respiration. Finally, the ether element is absorbed into the light.

As in many scriptures and traditional teachings, *The Tibetan Book of the Dead* affirms that the departed spirit first experiences a wondrous and compelling light. It appears that light is the initial manifestation of pure energy and is the first to be experienced upon the dissolution of the body. It is reported to be reassuringly beautiful.

Energy, it seems, has four intrinsic qualities: light and sound, followed by motion and residual form. This can be evidenced physically in a thermonuclear reaction. The first phenomenon to be seen ejecting from a nuclear explosion is a blinding light, followed by sound, then by motion in the shape of shock waves, and lastly as heat and the mushroom cloud as the residual form. On a macrocosmic scale, the modern Big Bang theory of physics postulates a similar cataclysmic explosion from which this universe was formed. Physicists conceptualize that eventually our universe will implode into itself and eventually return into a state of emptiness where time, space and matter are nonexistent.

In many religions and world mythologies, light signifies the manifestation of the divine presence or state wherein wholeness is present. In Taoism the Void denotes the source from which light and sound arose, the "vibrationless original," followed by all of creation and to which creation eventually returns. The Void does not refer to spacial "emptiness", but to an unmanifest creative capacity. This is a mystery. That it is blissful is reassuring because we are part of it.

Thus, at death the departed spirit faces the beckoning light, which it initially merges with, but cannot stay in. This is because of karmic conditioning that brings back the awareness of the soul as separate. The spiritual quest is to achieve union which dissolves the (negative) karmic requirement to be reborn. Then rebirths may happen by choice for a higher purpose. The soul whose evolution is incomplete may also fear what may arise from sensing the primal Void behind the light. In any case, after this stage there is a period referred to as the great swoon or disorientation, followed by the journey through the realms of disincarnate existence until the next rebirth. *The Tibetan Book of the Dead* is used to instruct the adept in the means by which he or she can merge with the light. If this fails, the person is then guided to an auspicious rebirth for continued spiritual growth. The spirit continually seeks form to wrap itself in; it does this voluntarily or by karmic necessity. Yet spirit is paramount and eternal. Spirit is fundamentally not dependent on the body, although modern science and medicine would have us believe precisely the opposite.

Most religions believe that human life is a precious gift and opportunity. Throughout the ages, mystics and sages have affirmed that human beings can potentially experience wholeness and a mystical union with life's source. Some, like the Buddhists, believe that only in a human incarnation can karma's momentum be altered or even extinguished, while karma's effects, good and bad, are reaped, both in this human existence and in other disincarnate forms of the spirit.

I am reminded of a story shared by one of my patients, Debbie. Her husband John had always been a materialist who did not believe in rebirth, afterlife, or a spiritual existence beyond the world of his senses. To his dismay, Debbie did believe in such things and frequently talked to their friends and others about her ideas. Indeed, she had considered herself a Buddhist for many years. Whenever she brought up one of her spiritual beliefs, John would get annoyed and upset, wishing she'd keep her ideas to herself, since he felt embarrassed by what he perceived as her misguided talk. John eventually contracted a kidney disorder which led to a progressive failure of the organs. As he approached death, they agreed that should he die, no attempt whatsoever was to be made to resuscitate him.

As it happened, John did die after being quite ill for some time. To the dismay of his wife, who had not been present, the hospital staff revived John and put him on life-support. Once Debbie found out what was happening, she became very upset and demanded that the hospital administration immediately stop using the machines that kept John alive, since this was against his express wishes. The hospital administration refused to take him off the machines for the first 24 hours, because they feared jeopardizing their hospital records. The next day, a few moments after the life-support machines were stopped, John suddenly awoke from his coma and said to his wife:

"Debbie, guess what, guess what? I was dead. It was more wonderful than anything that you have ever told anyone." John confessed that he did not want to stay in this world any longer; he wanted to go there into death. John and Debbie felt connected as never before. He died peacefully a few hours later. What a gift for him to come back and give this confirmation to her - something neither of them could ever have anticipated!

Exercise 2
Letting Go: The Dark Tunnel

The purpose of this visualization or guided imagery is to explore your life's meaning and how it would be if you were to let go of your present form. By doing this exercise, perhaps you will learn something about your inner self. Your true inner self is enjoyable. Invite it to be present. Remember to gently let the images, feelings, sensations and thoughts come as they may; do not hold on or resist the impressions that arise; they are after all a part of you. Honor them as you would your spirit.

Start by finding a comfortable place to relax. This exercise will take about 20 minutes. You may want to lie down or sit in an easy chair. Close your eyes and just notice your present state. After a few moments, begin letting go of any physical tension by breathing in and out. At the same time, let your thoughts be quieted and your feelings calmed as you continue to breathe.

Keeping your eyes closed, imagine that you have just died; your body is now inert, lifeless. Slowly your energy dissolves and you envision your spirit leaving the body. You are now in the room but outside your body, hovering over it. Looking down on your body you start to see your past; you behold the differing physical forms your body once had on life's journey. The adult, teen, child and infant form are remembered and with them the important life events that defined who you were. Good or bad, painful or joyous, traumatic or sublime, you accept them. Reflect on the inner meaning of your life. Let yourself remember what was important and imagine what thought, life lesson, or hope you could take from this life into the next.

In a few moments you sense a pull; you may even start to see a light. You feel as if you're entering a dark tunnel steadily moving toward the light that is straight ahead. You are being drawn away from this place, away from all that you once were, your body, identity, career, family, friends, possessions and responsibilities. All that you have ever known is about to be left behind. Ask yourself:

What does your spirit feel?
Am I ready for this journey?
If not, what still needs attending to?
What do I need to let go of?
What do I sense about the light?
Is there a sense of love in and around my spirit?

Give yourself time to reflect in this state, take in any messages and images that arise in your consciousness.

Now turn around in the tunnel and look back at your body. Notice that you are aware of breathing again, and slowly reenter and reintegrate with your body. Take a few deep breaths and sense your body.

You may want to reflect on anything that arose during this visualization. You can repeat this exercise whenever desired. You may find that inner clarity arises, as well as a new found direction and sense of gratitude.

C H A P T E R   T H R E E

The Psychoenergetic Core

*"Shape clay into a vessel; it is the space within
that makes it useful." - Lao Zi*

Often I have wandered in the labyrinth of my soul. I
have discovered patterns, images and memories I never
knew existed. Sometimes I have been pained at what I
found, and at other times overwhelming joy has bathed
my entire being upon some inner discovery. I sense there
is a possibility of infinite expression within me. Yet, I have
found a mysterious world inside myself that is profoundly orderly in nature. In this chapter, I will explore the
innermost reaches of this world, the psychoenergetic core.

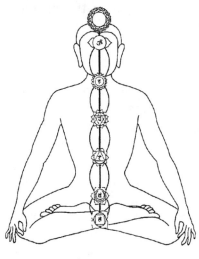

**3-1 Indian Sushumna-Chakras
   System**

This drawing illustrates the symbolic
form and envisioned location of the
seven major chakras along the
sushumna in the Indian tradition. The
psychoenergetic centers with their
Sanskrit name and associated element
or state in ascending order are:
1. Base - *Muladhara* - earth,
2. Vitality - *Svadhishthana* - water,
3. Solar - *Manipura* - fire,
4. Heart - *Anahata* - air,
5. Throat - *Vishudha* - ehter,
6. Brow - *Ajna* - primal duality
7. Crown - *Sahasrara* - transcendental

Human consciousness and the psychoenergetic core do not have a physical form, although they exist within the gross body. However, the core can be visualized as running vertically from the crown of the head to the perineum at the base of the pelvis. Along the core are seven distinctive centers, as has been described within the Indian concept of the sushumna-chakras. The seven centers from the top of the head to the perineum are as follows: the Crown, Brow, Throat, Heart, Solar, Vitality and Base. All of these centers will be individually discussed in the next chapter.

Each psychoenergetic center has a nucleus and surrounding field, just like an atomic structure. The nucleus stabilizes the causal and mental spheres while the surrounding field refracts consciousness outward into the surrounding physical and energetic structures. The field generates and fades into another energetic structure, the transverse currents, which I will discuss in Chapter 7 in detail. Together, nucleus and field form a Yin-Yang relationship, of concentration and diffusion. Proper balance within the psychoenergetic core depends on two factors: equilibrium between the nucleus and surrounding field and the vertical free flow and alignment of the centers along the psychoenergetic core.

Psychoenergetic Core's Functions

As mentioned, the psychoenergetic core primarily functions to orient and diffuse consciousness, which first appears with the incarnating soul. The vibrational frequency of the core becomes differentiated as the spirit grounds itself into the body. This occurs in a descending fashion within the core along seven stages, like the sequence in the musical scale. Thus, at each stage along the psychoenergetic core there is a different vibrational density or rate. The spirit's grounding into the physical is not complete until subtle cords or roots are anchored downward from the base center. This process occurs within the first years of life as the incarnating spirit identifies with the body, or establishes its effective occupancy.

I should explain here that vibrational frequencies are the subtle rates of oscillation or movement which occur in all phenomena. The waves at the subatomic level, such as at an atom's nucleus, vibrate 10^{22} times per second, while molecules vibrate at approximately 10^9 times per second. In comparison, the vibrational frequency of audible sound is extremely dense; for example, the lowest note on a piano pulses or vibrates at 27.5 beats per second, while the highest note vibrates at 4,186 beats per second.

During the infant's first years, while the spirit is not fully grounded, the infant's fontanel on the top of the head remains open. The downward grounding process and the closing of the fontanel occur synchronistically, over relatively the same period of time. The open fontanel is representative of the spirit's continued communion with the divine sphere.

The subtle roots at the Base center of the psychoenergetic core, besides anchoring the spirit, allow for the discharge of excess psychic energy via the body throughout life. Additionally, this grounding mechanism helps maintain the energetic and magnetic resonance between the physical body and the earth. In Taoism these cords are visualized as descending downwards through the pelvis and legs, extending to the soles of the feet.

According to many traditional teachings, the spirit or soul enters the physical body through the fontanel on the top of the head. This physical opening is referred to in Indian philosophy as the Gate of Brahma, the creator, and by the Chinese as the Heavenly gate. This gate is subtly perceptible in newborns as a vibration and pulsation. The bones of the skull eventually fill in the soft fontanel and completely cover the openings by about the end of the first year. Physically, in the womb, the embryo develops from the umbilicus outward and generally upward towards the head. During the metamorphic months of pregnancy, life-sustaining and life-building substances enter from the mother through the umbilical cord. Similarly, the psychoenergetic core is originally formed as an energetic space within the nascent embryo's tissues, near the site of the future navel.

After birth, the infant's awareness matures sequentially from above to below, from the head downward. Each center along the psychoenergetic core progressively facilitates awareness to develop and consciousness to organize itself. In time, this awareness will lead to nerve control over the biological structures. During infancy the baby first learns to control and utilize the eyes and mouth, while at the same time sounds are recognized and produced. The head during this period appears proportionately larger than the body. Slowly the motor functions of the neck become easier to command, followed by the arms and hands. Next the spine becomes firm and lower legs manageable, and crawling and walking skills are mastered. Lastly the excretory reflexes are brought under control.

On the other hand, human beings grow and mature psychologically in the course of a lifetime in the reverse order to physical development. That is to say, the accessible psychological contents of the psychoenergetic centers are naturally integrated in an ascending fashion, from the lowest center at the base of the perineum upwards. The key word here is accessible, since usually the personality becomes arrested at different levels, due to the karmic restraints of the psyche.

Heaven, Earth and Humanity

In classical Chinese philosophy the concept of heaven, earth and humanity offers a powerful metaphor for understanding the relationships within the psychoenergetic core and the human being as a whole. Specifically, the head is associated with heaven, the cosmos. The heaven is considered Yang, being the seat of the creative potential and the abode of the spirit. The earth is opposite to heaven. Earth is visualized as encompassing the abdomen, and by extension the lower limbs which ground us to the physical world. The earth is considered Yin, a yielding and receptive force from which all biological life arises. The biological matrix and reproductive seed of life, called "essence" in Chinese philosophy, originates and develops from within the abdomen. The essence, like the earth, is the fundamental building block and means for physical development.

Between heaven and earth is the level of humanity, as represented by the chest region in the human body. In Chinese medicine the breast bone is called the central altar, signifying the place from which one can venerate both heaven and earth. The area of the chest, being neutral in polarity, incorporates the forces of both Yin and Yang. Qi, which can be viewed as a potential generated by Yin and Yang, is centered in and moves out through the chest. The hands are sometimes considered an extension

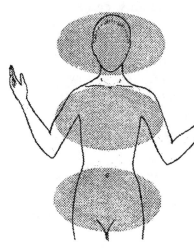

3-2 Heaven, Earth and Humanity

This figure shows the three classical divisions of the human form according to Chinese philosophy. They are in ascending order

1. *Earth* in compassing the abdomen, pelvis and legs, 2. *Humanity* which embraces the heart, chest and arms, and 3. *Heaven* or cosmos which relates to the head and neck region.

of this level, since through the hands we can easily express our Qi.

Similarly, a natural polarization also occurs within the psychoenergetic core, along a vertical axis between the Crown and Base centers. The Heart center is the fulcrum, functioning as both a regulator and capacitor, to accumulate an energetic charge for the system. Above the Heart center each center is progressively more Yang in polarity; while downward from the Heart center the Yin becomes predominant.

The Base and Crown respectively form the Yin and Yang poles of the psychoenergetic core, along the vertical axis. Yet they do not contain absolute states of polarization, since Yin and Yang cannot exist in isolation. In traditional thought all things contain some form of duality, as represented by Yin and Yang, in subtle or gross form. Principally, the Crown and Base centers function as gates or barriers for restraining the movement of psychic contents within the psychoenergetic core. These two centers retain latent psychic energy and are normally dormant, activated only at the transitions of birth, death or upon a spiritual awakening of the individual.

The Vitality and Brow centers, for their part, manifest greater functional activity. The Vitality center, like the Base, is Yin in polarity while the Brow, as the Crown, is more Yang in polarity. Equally important in functional activity is the Heart center, which is the neutral fulcrum between the polarized Vitality and the Brow centers. Hence, the Vitality and Brow centers are the active poles within the psychoenergetic core, while the Base and Crown centers manifest the passive poles.

The Three Divisions in the Tibetan System

In the Tibetan system we find aspects of both the Chinese and Indian teachings. Lama Govinda, in his book

Foundations of Tibetan Mysticism, explains that the Tibetans divide the Buddhist five-chakra system into three divisions or zones: the upper zone (stod) or cosmic plane, to which the two centers of the Brow and Throat belong; a middle zone (bar) or human plane, to which the Heart center belongs; and a lower zone (smad) or earth plane, to which the Solar and Vitality centers belong. He goes on to explain that the upper and lower zones form a polarity, while the Heart center mediates between them. Strangely, in the Buddhist system the Crown and Base centers do not play a significant role. About the zones themselves Lama Govinda says:

"These three zones represent in their deepest sense:

1. The terrestrial plane, namely the earth-bound elementary forces of nature, of materiality or corporeality (of the materialized past);

2. The cosmic or universal plane of eternal laws, of timeless knowledge (which from the human point of view is felt as a 'future' state of attainment, a goal yet to be attained), a plane of spontaneous spiritual awareness of the Infinite, as symbolized in the boundlessness of space and in the experience of the Great Void, in which form and non-form are equally comprised;

3. The human plane of individual realization, in which the qualities of terrestrial existence and cosmic relationship, the forces of the earth and of the universe become conscious in the human soul as an ever-present and deeply felt reality."

The Tibetan teachings on the three aspects or zones within human beings are not unique; in both the Chinese and Indian traditions we find similar concepts. More specifically, in the Taoist teachings the three Fields of

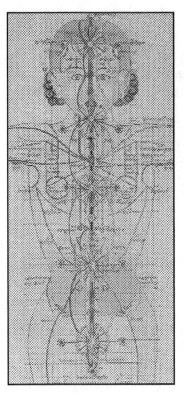

3-3 Tibetan Chakra Figure

This authoritative drawing from the *Blue Beryl*, treatise of Sangye Gyamtso (1653 - 1705 A.D.), illustrates the Tibetan Buddhist view of the chakras (*rsta-khor*) and sushumna (*dbu-ma*). This tradition emphasizes the existence of five major chakras which are depicted possessing twenty-four spokes said to symbolize their ability to generate and link with the numerous subtle meridians or currents (*rsta*). The Brow and Throat centers are associated with the cosmic plane (*stod*), the Heart center to the human plane (*bar*), and the Solar and Vitality centers to the earth plane (*smad*).

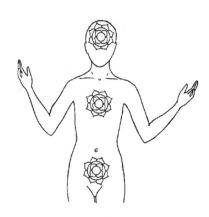

Influence (dan tian) correspond to the Brow, Heart, and Vitality centers, while in the Hindu Tantric tradition the same three centers are referred to as the three Knots (granthi). Through the Brow, Heart and Vitality centers the core can be most easily accessed and influenced. Also, at these centers karmic restrictions are more profound in nature.

3-4 Knots, Zones and Fields of Influence

The Brow, Heart and Vitality centers are the focal points for the mental, energetic and physical spheres, respectively. In the Orient, these centers are referred to under different names and images yet their meaning reveal a convergent understanding. The Chinese concept of the three Fields of Influence concurs with the Indian idea of the three Knots (the Brow, Heart, and Vitality centers).

Fundamentally the Brow center is the gravitational pole of the mental sphere, the Heart center is the focus of the energetic sphere (especially the meridian system and aura, which I will discuss later) and the Vitality center is the hub of the physical sphere.

Sound

The psychoenergetic core envelops and orients the causal and mental spheres. On the fundamental level, light and sound are the residual forms of energy that remain within the core immediately before physical death. Light and sound are essential attributes of the refined consciousness that inhabits the causal sphere. This inner or sacred light and sound is beyond our ordinary perception. However, in my experience, visible light and audible sound can be used as pathways towards the unseen and unheard realm of pure awareness and energy.

During the period of embodied life, all four intrinsic aspects of pure energy manifest within the psychoenergetic core. Light, sound, motion and residual form appear within the core in a descending order from the most subtle or refined to denser quality. The Brow center is linked with cosmic light, energy's most refined manifestation, the Heart and Throat centers with cosmic sound, and the Solar center with spontaneous vibration manifesting energy's motion. The Base and Vitality centers are associated with mystic heat, pure energy's residual form. The Crown center is considered the source of pure energy, the unknowable Void.

Divine sound is referred to in India as shabda and in China as gong. This primordial sound has been theoretically linked to the universe's background "noise", which originated from the cosmic Big Bang and is now a diffused resonance throughout the universe.

In a way, audible sound is an extension of the sacred sound that is associated with the psychoenergetic core. Fundamentally sound is composed of three attributes: pulse, wave and form. Pulse is the power behind both wave and form. Wave refers to motion, while form signifies manifestation. Like Yin and Yang, they are complementary and inter-dynamic, existing always together with the unitary pulse as their root.

Dr. Hans Jenny, the developer of Cymatics (the study of the inter-relationship of wave-form and matter) has photographed sound through an instrument he developed, known as the tonoscope. These images strikingly resemble mandalas and geometric formations (called yantras in Sanskrit). Sound, when projected through the tonoscope (that uses various solid or liquid mediums), produces surprising images. Jenny proved that sound when visually translated will produce a geometric form. Interestingly, Albert Einstein visualized matter as being like an excited state of "dynamic geometry."

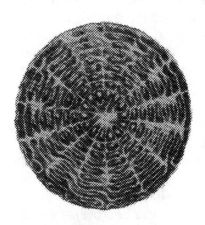

3-5 Cymatic Photograph

According to Dr. Jenny's experiments using a tonoscope sound vibrations can be sculptured into visible form through physical mediums such as sand, powder, liquid, and metal filings. The photograph reveals the manifestation of audible sound when projected onto a plate of fine lycopodium powder. Sound was electronically generated via oscillation crystals in this experiment.

According to Jenny's research the Indian mantra Om generates the form of the Sri Yantra on the tonoscope. Om is representative of the cosmic sound. It is a monosyllabic word formed by the combination of three sounds: a, u, and m, which are used to denote the three evolutionary phases of the cosmic cycle (creation, preservation and destruction). The ancient rishis of India tell us that the Sri Yantra is the manifest form of that very same sound, Om. What was once strictly an internal mystic insight is now, via modern scientific technique, a reproducible phenomenon.

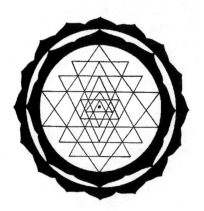

3-6 Sri Yantra

This sacred symbol and meditation device is said to represent the cosmic field of creation that contains the polarized forces of generation and destruction. The central dot (*bindu*) is the seat of the primal sound *OM* which binds together and harmonizes the contesting forces in their primary form.

Personally, I have been graced with the experience of perceiving the inner yantras, of various designs, that exist within the centers of the psychoenergetic core. They manifest in a host of shapes and colors and are wondrous to behold.

Light

Both sound and light are perceived to organize themselves naturally into a sequential order of seven, as in the seven colors of the rainbow and the seven-note major scale. Furthermore, sound frequencies are slower than light. Yet, according to the Law of Octaves, a specific sound can be translated into color of a like frequency. The Law of Octaves states that the eighth note repeats the first note via the seven-note scale, but at double the vibrational frequency. For example, in singing the syllables of the major scale "do, re, mi, fa, sol, la, te, do", the second do is one octave higher than the first. It has been estimated that a leap of forty octaves is needed to move from the audible sound waves to the visible light waves that produce color. Middle C (256 cycles per second) approximates the visible color red, according to the Law of Octaves. In fact, the whole spectrum of irradiated energy - including x-rays, light, heat, radio waves, visible color and so on - covers a range of about seventy octaves.

As stated above, light and sound are two attributes of pure energy. The other two are motion and residual form. Light and sound are higher in frequency, while motion and form are more dense. Light travels faster then sound and, unlike sound, does not need air through which to move. I perceive that pure light and sound are like the pulse, the primal force, while both wave (motion) and form are extensions of light and sound. The various centers along the psychoenergetic core have been linked to the seven-fold patterns of visible light and audible sound as follows:

CENTER	COLOR	NOTE
Crown	violet	B
Brow	indigo	A
Throat	blue	G
Heart	green	F
Solar	yellow	E
Vitality	orange	D
Base	red	C

I must give a word of caution; the various associations and attributes associated with the psychoenergetic centers, as listed above and elsewhere, should be considered as relative and not firm linkages. As I have mentioned previously, individual differences of psychoenergetic expression occur naturally, as surely as DNA varies amongst human beings. We can also find, from culture to culture or from age to age within a culture, variations in the perceived color, sound, and attributes of a center. Perhaps this is so because mankind's innate perception of sound evolves with awareness and consciousness. For example, physically, in the history of musical tuning, during Beethoven's time the tuning was much lower, over half a step of difference; his Pastoral Symphony in F Major would sound higher today, similar to F# major. Therefore, in studying the energetic terrain I have emphasized general pattern because the system is by nature dynamic, not static. Culturally many variations result from "free choice" and the ability to condition "tastes."

The power of sacred music and sound, in the form of mantras and prayer, has long been regarded as a powerful tool for spiritual awakening and healing. The mind and body seem to be able to amplify sound as well as being able to absorb and attenuate colors and other subtle vibrations; all of this can affect the individual's energetic terrain. How far these external influences reach into the energetic structure and psychoenergetic core is perhaps dependent on the overall openness of the person and auspiciousness of the moment. I believe that there are always synchronistic factors involved with any spontaneous awakening or expansion of the forces within the energetic terrain.

Archetypal Images

Psychologically, each center contains specific archetypal images and functions of both a personal and collective nature. These centers hold a highly complex and manifold set of impressions, from the transcendental to the mundane, in symbolic image form. The individual centers along the core can be seen as representing a journey toward psychological wholeness, which in Jungian terms closely parallels the individuation process.

Each specific center along the psychoenergetic core represents configurations within the psyche, composed of transpersonal and personal infraconscious material, as well as projections of the conscious mind. The personal infraconscious acts as an intermediary between the conscious mind and the transpersonal infraconscious. The personal infraconscious primarily functions as a storehouse for thoughts not yet ripe for consciousness, lost or repressed memories, or subliminal perceptions that contain impressions of past events. These in turn condition the individual's karmic patterns.

The transpersonal infraconscious, on the other hand, contains the whole inherited wealth of humanity's psychological evolution. Expression of the transpersonal infraconscious appears to be in the form of primordial, mythological and spiritual images. This is also the source of genuine creativity and the womb of future thought processes.

The conscious mind, which includes the ego, can infiltrate the psychoenergetic core. The conscious mind forms our awareness of individuality in terms of our physical body, emotions, personality, and thoughts. The conscious mind enjoys an illusion of autonomy separate from the infraconscious realms, because it is capable of misinterpreting and distorting perceptions of reality. This is done for its own survival and is achieved by repressing unwanted memories and desires into the personal infraconscious. Thereafter these patterns become part of the contents of a center along the psychoenergetic core. This is why the ego aspect of the mind may become terrified or threatened when contact is made with the contents of the core.

The great sages all emphasize the virtues of unconditional love and compassion because they assist the aspirant in the inward journey. Love and compassion free the ego restraints of consciousness, thus allowing the psychoenergetic centers to be awakened gently and without threat to the mind.

Exercise 3
Finding the Core

The psychoenergetic core lies deep within us all. It silently orders our mind and spirit, both the conscious and infraconscious aspects. In this visualization you will try to localize this structure within your self.

Find a comfortable and quiet place to sit or lie down. Keep your back relatively straight and relaxed with your arms and legs uncrossed. You will need about 15 - 20 minutes to complete this exercise. Close your eyes and start by concentrating upon your breath. Follow the inhalation and exhalation phases. Let any intrusive thoughts, feelings and sensations melt away as you follow the breath. Continue breathing slowly and deeply.

Begin by visualizing a fine threadlike structure running from the top of your head to the perineum (between the anus and the genital organs). Perhaps you will find that this core structure has a color. If not, imagine a soft golden light emanating from the core. As you breathe in, allow energy progressively to rise up in the threadlike core from the perineum to the top of your head. Let it fill the core like water fills a vessel. Now, when you breathe out imagine energy sinking down the threadlike core from the top of the head to the perineum. Follow this up and down motion, and allow your breathing and visualization to become integrated and fluid in motion. As this happens, slowly shift your focus to the energy and less upon the actual motion of the breath. In this way, follow the movement of subtle energy along the core for about 5 - 10 minutes.

When you have finished, slowly open your eyes and relax for a minute before moving. Take this time to reflect on your experience. Often people have deep insights into their inner nature when they perform this exercise. It is a helpful technique to center yourself when stressed or to get in touch with your vital energy.

C H A P T E R   F O U R

Seven Oceans

*"Within this earthen vessel are seven oceans and
innumerable stars." - Kabir*

Throughout history different individuals and societies
have used compelling images to describe their insights
and knowledge of the psychoenergetic core. In the above
quote, the psychoenergetic centers are called oceans by
Kabir, the Indian mystic. The word ocean symbolically
connotes a primal mystery of profound depth. It has often
struck me that we call our planet "the earth" in spite of
the fact that the terrestrial oceans account for about three
quarters of this planet's surface. Those magnificent pho-
tos from space showing an overwhelmingly blue planet
demonstrate how vital the oceans are to planetary life.

Similarly, within ourselves is another primal mystery
in the form of seven centers, each with its unique expression. Like the oceans, the psychoenergetic centers are distinct, yet connected by subtle currents of energy that flow
between them. The disc-like mandala representations of
the centers depicted in classical texts reveal this awareness of individual integrity at each station along the core.

Once, many years ago when I was in my teens, I
attended a gathering with some native friends on the
coast of California. I participated in the ceremonies and
partook in the ritual use of a sacred plant, peyote. The day

was glorious and after a time when the ceremonies had ended and the effects of the plant seemed dissipated, I wandered off alone into the nearby redwood forest to rest and gather myself. Somehow I found myself by an ancient tree that had an opening at its base. The opening was about three feet high and about two feet wide. I looked inside and found, to my surprise, a small space that was just big enough for my body to comfortably fit in. I felt an overwhelming urge to crawl right in, so I did. As I sat there cross legged, I noticed that above my head the darkened space seem to extend upwards for some distance, perhaps a dozen yards. I closed my eyes and immediately I sensed a great relaxation bathe my entire body and mind. For a moment, I imagined that I was in a kind of grandmother tree and that I was nestled in her womb. Soon I fell into a light trance in which I began to connect with and sense the energy of the tree. Slowly I perceived a breath-like movement of energy going up and down my body. At first I thought it was the tree that was doing this to me; moments later I realized that this force was actually internal and gently pushing my breath up and down, in and out. This was my life force, not the tree's; the tree had shown me the way inside. I focused on the force and began to perceive a subtle background energy behind it; my awareness descended into a bright tunnel along which were different levels or centers filled with extraordinary images. How long I stayed there, I do not know. I was completely absorbed in this inner world and nothing else seemed to exist. Then a curious thing happened; I noticed that my breathing had slowed right down to almost a standstill; it was only faintly present. I sensed an overwhelming urge to breathe and at once I reentered my normal mind-body awareness. So ended one of my first conscious encounters with the psychoenergetic core.

In the following pages I would like to share my understanding of the psychoenergetic core and its seven centers. Remember, this outline of the centers is but a reference point, revealing their primary features. In reality, every individual has a unique configuration within his or her psychoenergetic centers, just as one's experience of them is bound to be unique.

Base Center

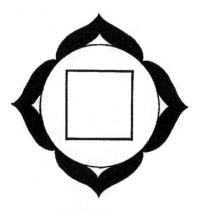

4-1 Base Image

The Base center is the passive Yin pole of the psychoenergetic core. Intuitively viewed, this center resides in front of the base of the spine and near the perineum. Interestingly, the Chinese word for perineum, huiyin, can be literally translated as the meeting of Yin.

There are three classical symbols that can give us insight into the nature of a psychoenergetic center. They consist of an image of petals, an allied element, and geometric design. In Tantric texts, a center's vibrational frequency is traditionally depicted by a distinctive set of petals. Elemental affinity not only corresponds with a center's vibrational frequency, but also gives us a clue about its special qualities, while geometric design gives us a hint about its dynamic function.

Classical texts assign to the Base center four petals. The concept of four is frequently used in primitive cultures to aid in orientation, for example in the quartering of the world into four directions, an idea that appears within very diverse cultures, from China to Europe to the native peoples of the Americas.

Four also is an emblem for the mind's way to orient itself. Dr. Carl Jung refers to this as the quaternity motif which has appeared in many forms throughout history, such as: a) in cultural images like the mandala, square or cross; b) in the fundamental modes of perception: thinking, feeling, sensing and moving; c) in archaic world-views, as the ancient Greek model of the four elements: earth, water, fire and air; or the medical theories of Hippocrates (460 - 370 BC) and Galen (129 - 200 AD), in which the four humors of blood, phlegm, black and yellow bile were used to differentiate human temperaments; and d) in science one speaks of four natural constants: energy, gravitation, affinity, and weak interaction, or of Einstein's four-dimensional model of the universe.

In terms of elemental affinity, the Base center is linked to the earth. In Indian philosophy there are five representative elements which have differing levels of vibrational activity. From lowest to highest, they are earth, water, fire, air, and ether. The two centers in the head are beyond the domain of these material elements. The Base center, associated with the earth, occupies the lowest position in terms of vibrational density, which is reflected in its compact field of resonance and ability to ground the spirit to the physical form.

The geometric symbol of the Base center is the square. The square represents the ability of the spirit to integrate itself with its physical existence. Furthermore, the square denotes this center's function of stabilizing the whole psychoenergetic core. In fact, the literal meaning of the Base center's Sanskrit name, muladhara, is foundation.

An important function of this center is to store a latent primordial potential, which is referred to as the kundalini or original Qi, respectively, in Tantra and Taoism. Kundalini (or kundalini shakti) literally means the energy of the coiled feminine serpent. The kundalini, or feminine serpent, which routinely sheds her skin, mythologically represents the soul's enclosure in form, time and space. The arousal of the kundalini is classically expressed by the image of a snake uncoiling herself and rising upwards. This same energy is referred to by Lao Zi, the founder of Taoism, as the mysterious female. The functions of the kundalini are in my opinion twofold: to facilitate the grounding of spirit and the suppression of past life memories.

I should point out that at each center along the psychoenergetic core, karmic patterns are contained which have an effect upon the psyche and energetic terrain. An awakening within a center generates subtle changes according to its established karmic patterns. At each center, sound, color and form, as well as the release of mystic heat and kinetic energy, may be experienced as part of a changing inner awareness.

Specifically, the Base center tends to entrap past life memories. Contacting and awakening this center will initiate the reemergence of dormant images and thoughts, especially memories of previous births and deaths, important past life events, spiritual awakenings, and other momentous experiences. Most likely, past life memories are suppressed by the latent kundalini's inertia.

In both Taoism and Tantra the arousal and ascent of the kundalini is of paramount concern. This is because the arousal of the kundalini loosens the connection between consciousness and matter, thereby freeing the individual to experience higher states of awareness and to integrate karmic patterns that reach far back into past lives.

Often the initial manifestation of kundalini awakening is accompanied by an experience of intense heat. This phenomenon has been called the spiritual baptism of fire. Awakening the kundalini also produces a progressive intensification of the vibrational frequency of the centers, which in turn adds potency to the kundalini's force. This process liberates the karmic constraints and patterns found within the centers. Although this process usually begins within the Base center, there is no fixed sequence of events thereafter, as the kundalini awakens the centers above the Base.

Depending upon a person's karma, the awakening of the Base center and its contained kundalini can happen gradually or suddenly, and it can be intensely or subtly noticeable. As the kundalini becomes activated, all the centers along the core undergo change. Symbolically viewed, this change occurs along a vertical direction, from below upwards, within the core. However, the integration of the psychic contents of each center is equally important, a process which I view as an expansion or lateral movement within a center's mandala-like structure. Ideally, balanced spiritual growth consists of progress in both vertical and lateral directions.

Psychologically, the three lower centers below the Heart tend to manifest more personal infraconscious patterns of mind, which are normally below the threshold of memory. In contrast, the three higher centers above the Heart mainly embrace aspects of the transpersonal infraconscious. The Heart center primarily facilitates the integration of the infraconscious, in both its personal and transpersonal aspects. Nevertheless, each center contains a portion of all aspects of the psyche; only the emphasis of its contents varies.

Furthermore, the Base center is closely linked with instinctual patterns of survival, whether they be mental, emotional or physical. Ideally, when a person has experienced a relatively calm, nurturing and healthy gestation, birth and early infancy, as well as a strong primal bonding with the mother and father, his or her inner need for security and nurturing should have been satisfied. If this did not happen, the Base center may have become blocked and one's personality arrested at the survival level of consciousness. The natural urge to grow, consume and learn in infancy and childhood are a healthy reflection of the spirit's desire and ability to survive.

Vitality Center

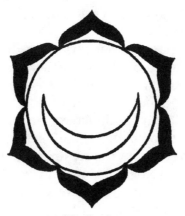

4-2 Vitality Image

The Vitality center forms the active Yin pole of the psychoenergetic core. It is perceived to be located within the lower abdomen, slightly anterior to the sacral bone. In Taoism, this center is called the Lower Field of Influence. I find that through this center consciousness learns to deal with the biological demands of being incarnate. The Vitality center constitutes one of the three Knots where subtle energy can easily become concentrated, as well as blocked; the other two Knots are the Heart and Brow centers.

The Vitality center is classically represented by the crescent moon, its geometric symbol. The earth's moon, with its monthly cycles of waxing and waning, expresses the image of the procreative potential. In many traditional cultures the moon is linked to the reproductive cycle and the flow of energy within the body. It affects tides and their rhythms, and, physiologically, periods of fertility in men and women, the brain's activity, and so forth. The Vitality center is associated with the water element, which of course the moon influences. In figurative terms, the Base and Vitality centers complement each others' nature. This is expressed as follows: earth without water would be lifeless and water without earth would have no form to contain it.

This center's name in Sanskrit is svadhishthana, literally meaning one's own abode. I believe that through this center, identification with one's body occurs. While the Base center grounds consciousness, it is through the Vitality center that consciousness becomes functionally connected to the body. As we shall see in the next chapter, the Vitality center is closely linked to the motivational center of embryological growth. The Vitality center is represented by six petals, one level of vibrational frequency above the Base center.

In addition, the physical area around this center is biomechanically considered the body's center of gravity. As mentioned earlier, the mental, energetic and physical spheres have their operative seat respectively within the Brow, Heart and Vitality centers. Nevertheless, the mental and energetic spheres are both anchored to the physical body through the Vitality center.

I imagine the Vitality center to function like an alchemical cauldron in which the forces of polarization are reconciled. Psychologically, this polarization is sexual in nature, in the form of the anima and animus archetypes, to use the Jungian terms. At this center the primal motivation of the psyche is to merge the male and female duality. On a most fundamental level this is a process of reconciling the feminine and masculine forces. When the inner forces are reconciled, one's spirit, mind and energy experiences a blissful union which is accompanied by a powerful syntonic feeling of oneness throughout the physical body. The syntonic feeling is one of intimate connection to oneself and to all of life surrounding us. This profound desire for a union of the anima-animus within oneself is however most commonly expressed, in our awareness, as a sexual urge directed externally.

In adolescence the awakening of sexuality occurs naturally. Unfortunately, the conscious mind filters and distorts (because of its own latent karma or recently acquired impressions) the primal desire for inner union, only to seek outward union with an appropriate female or male partner. For each individual, his or her predominating inner sexual identification will be attracted to the inner sexual identity of a desired partner. Vibrationally, like attracts like, whether balanced or distorted. Inner sexual identity is determined by our own reconciliation of the male and female duality. Thus the physical gender of two people may be different or the same depending upon their inner identification. This is perhaps the reason why there is such a variety of sexual preference amongst human beings.

Indeed, the combination of karmic tendencies, including psychological and physical traumas, often results in a distorted view of sexual functioning. Recognizing the underlying character of the sexual urge is an important evolutionary step along the path of spiritual and psychological growth. In a society where sexual addiction and dysfunction, as well as codependence between mates, is commonplace, we must seriously look within this center for understanding.

Solar Center

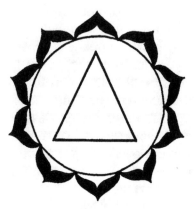

4-3 Solar Image

The Solar center is associated with the fire element and the geometric flame-like triangle symbol. The traditional Sanskrit name of this center, manipur, signifying gem center, also suggests a radiant quality. While the Base center represents earth's solidity and the Vitality center water's fluidity, the Solar center embodies the idea of fire's transformative quality. This center is fundamentally dynamic in nature. Classically, ten petals are used to denote its vibrational quality. The Solar center can be visualized as residing within the abdomen, slightly above and posterior to the physical navel.

This center is the focus through which both internal and external resonances are assimilated and transformed. From an energetic perspective, external resonances are subtly and continually taken in through the body's navel, paralleling the way the navel once absorbed the physical nutrients during its embryological stage of life. Externally, environmental influences (from plants, animals, and people) and cosmic influences (from the sun, moon, stars, and so on) are mainly absorbed through the navel. Internally, the Solar center assimilates and transforms mental and energetic resonances from within the human being.

Psychologically, the Solar center represents a powerful transitional stage between the deep personal infraconscious realm of the lower centers and the potential for integration of the infraconscious in the Heart center. Powerful emotions or overwhelming mental and/or emotional stress will tend to first disturb the area around the Solar center. Anger, frustration, worry and excitement are especially disruptive to the expansive and free flowing nature of the forces found within this area. Interestingly, in many traditional cultures volcanoes are seen as earth's functional equivalent of the human body's navel. Physical shaking and cathartic reactions of the body often accompany the release of psychological and energetic restrictions that are within or around this center.

The Vitality and Base centers, in contrast, are linked with insufficiency states of the psyche: fear, insecurity, the compelling sexual desire, and most profoundly, the fear of death. All of these emotions are usually of a primordial quality that often serves as a basis for the more complex patterns associated with the Solar center.

Within life's journey the Solar center is linked to the development of personal power and the accumulation of knowledge. This normally is the pre-occupation of adulthood. With personal power comes an assertive tendency accompanied by a healthy sense of responsibility and desire to master one's abilities, while negatively it shows up as a desire to conquer and subjugate others or one's environment.

Collectively the three lower centers represent the instinctual urges and raw emotions that often possess human beings. Without any restraining force or spiritual awareness, these tendencies can be devastating. A human being's appreciation of the sanctity, oneness and wonder of life arises when the self has become liberated from the compulsion to act upon the primal urges. In this way true freedom of choice can be attained.

Heart Center

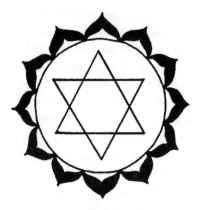

4-4 Heart Image

In the Indian tradition the name of the Heart center is anahata, meaning unstruck, referring to the "soundless" or sacred sound that is said to be heard within this center. In Taoism this center is called the Middle Field of Influence. In Tantra this is the site of the middle Knot. The Heart center acts like a fulcrum or pivot within the core; being situated halfway between the Crown and the Base centers, it is respectively referred to as heaven above and earth below. The Heart center is imagined as residing in the center of the physical chest.

The Heart center's function is to harmonize the psychoenergetic core, as much as a person's karmic restraints will allow. The Heart center's geometric symbol is the six-pointed star composed of two conjoined triangles. This star formation denotes integration and balance, the union of heaven and earth, the energies above and below this center. The Heart is denoted by twelve petals, which is equal to the number of outer points plus inner crossing points of the six pointed star formation. Twelve suggests that its vibrational frequency is not only high but also harmoniously balanced.

Through the Heart center the contents of the infraconscious, including the "shadow" within, can be integrated. The shadow, a psychological term, refers to the hidden or personal infraconscious aspects of oneself, both good and bad, which the ego has repressed or never recognized. Personal forgiveness and compassion should ideally accompany the infraconscious mind's illumination to consciousness of a higher order. In doing so, they facilitate the acceptance and eventual integration of the personal infraconscious into this level of conscious awareness. This process of illumination occurs on a deep personal level and is often followed by a peaceful outward identification with other fellow human beings and their suffering, and the desire to help, heal, and uplift.

In essence, the Heart center is where the percolation of the infraconscious aspects of mind comes to the surface. At this center both the personal and transpersonal aspects of the infraconscious are accessible, allowing ripened thoughts and images to be made available to the conscious mind. In this way they may potentially become integrated and used as expressive patterns of order, harmony, and beauty.

The Heart center is closely associated with the dream realm. Looking at the psychoenergetic core as a whole, the Brow center focuses our ordinary wakeful awareness within the brain. In other words, we usually sense and think from our head. When sleep becomes necessary, the awake mind is drawn downwards into the Throat center. Then the light and restless transitional stage of sleep begins as one's wakeful awareness dissolves. Next, when the Heart center receives the focus of mind, we enter a deeper sleep wherein the true dreaming state is found. Finally, the mind descends into the Solar and lower centers, allowing deep dreamless sleep to occur. Specifically, the Solar center assimilates any residual thoughts, while normal awareness is more-or-less suspended, as the body rejuvenates itself.

Generally, within the dreaming portion of sleep there are two important periods: the initial dream period after falling asleep and the pre-awakening dream period, usually before dawn. The initial dream period, when consciousness descends through the Throat and Heart centers, is mostly concerned with the digestion of the accumulated mental impressions from the day's experiences. On the other hand, the pre-awakening dream period closely reflects the infraconscious realms that are emerging as the focus of mind ascends through the Heart and Throat centers. The images and content of this pre-awakening dream period are of greater significance for understanding the deeper realms of the mind and its emerging patterns. However, gaining awareness of this dream realm generally requires practice and insight. The key for recalling one's dreams or remaining aware (lucid) while dreaming is to focus one's attention on the Throat center while falling asleep. Affirmations and visualizations are helpful in this regard.

Interestingly, the Indian rishis tell us that the mental sphere is tied to the physical body at the Heart center by a mystical silver cord. The function of this cord is to maintain a connection between one's mind and the physical body, should consciousness be willingly or unwillingly projected outside the body. This is called astral traveling, which can happen during meditation, trance states, sleep or in a host of other situations.

Anesthesia can also produce this same type of mind-body separation. Interestingly, there are surgical patients who have reported being fully or partially aware during an operation, as if they saw and heard what was happening in the operating room. Apparently, during these times the connection between the anesthetized physical body and wandering mind is maintained by this mysterious cord, rooted to the Heart center. A near-death experience may afford a similar out-of-body experience.

The Heart center is linked to the Air element, including the capacity to breathe. We cannot live physically without air, and it is from air that Qi (in the form of oxygen and other refined components) is absorbed by the lungs. The Heart center is connected to this process. Moreover, the Heart center closely resonates with the energetic sphere outside the core, especially the meridian system in which Qi circulates. More will be said about this in the coming chapters.

Psychologically, the Heart center is associated with the feelings of love, compassion and joy, whether personal or universal in sentiment. Forgiveness, as a certain attitude, and desire for goodwill which can awaken these noble feelings, is also linked with the Heart center.

On the other hand, grief, the loss of love or love's object, is particularly restrictive to vital energy flow around this center. Under the sway of this center, the stirring of love and desire for union can be felt for another person. The bonding desire between two people first occurs within this center, although it is often mixed up with the arousal of the procreative forces governed by the Vitality center. Nevertheless, the Heart center can transform the primal urges of the Vitality center into a more complete experience.

Along life's inner journey, the Heart center is where the lower center's urges and primal tendencies may be transformed and reconciled in love and compassion with one's higher spiritual purpose. An awakening of the Heart center happens when the self centeredness of mind surrenders to unconditional love. The trials and tribulations of marriage and family are great opportunities to delve into the depths of love, forgiveness and compassion. This period of life is an ideal time to awaken the Heart center and integrate its blessings.

Throat Center

4-5 Throat Image

The Throat center is linked to the ether element, which is an emblem for space. At this juncture along the core, the true expansiveness of consciousness is first sensed.

While earth is symbolized by a square, ether is geometrically represented by a circle. The circle, psychologically speaking, is symbolic of wholeness and integration in the psyche. In Chinese symbolism the ethers are the passageway to enter the heavenly abode.

The Throat center has 16 petals associated with it. The number 16, linked to the Throat center and ether, has as its square root 4, which denotes the Base center and earth element; thus there is also a quantitative relationship between the lowest and highest of the centers linked with the five elements. It is noteworthy that this even number sequence among the petals (4,6,10,12,16) is symbolic of the bipolar nature of reality.

This center is perceived to be located within the posterior part of the neck, above the level of the Adam's apple. The Sanskrit term for this center, visuddha, signifies cleansing and suggests that here purified awareness can be accessed.

Functionally the Throat center is affiliated with communication. Through releasing entrapped psychic energy within this center, consciousness begins to experience new realms of awareness. The transpersonal infraconscious is made available. Some mystics link the Throat center to the ability to access the so-called akashic records, the universal depository of all thoughts past and present (traditionally linked to the center of space), which is somewhat akin to the transpersonal infraconscious. However, to know the personal past one must uncover the latent memories stored within the Base center.

Musical creativity and inspired thinking are connected to the Throat center. The psychic faculty of clairaudience (the intuitive ability to hear inner messages and voices) can manifest itself through this center. Interestingly, physical impairment of hearing does not interfere with the ability to develop this psychic ability; in fact, deaf people are often naturally clairaudient.

In Ayurvedic philosophy, the faculty of hearing is associated with ether. For the most part, listening is a more passive sensory function than seeing, while together they form a complementary pair. Hearing is said to be the first sense awareness to develop in the fetus/newborn and is the last to leave before death.

Psychologically, this center facilitates the ability of the mind to articulate and express emotions and thoughts. Chronic inabilities to express oneself often manifest themselves as energetic restrictions in the neck, which is this center's sphere of influence.

In Chinese medicine the neck is a major transitional zone between the trunk of the body and the head. In classical acupuncture there exists in the neck the 'Windows of the Sky' points, which are able to liberate blocked Qi within this center's energetic area of influence. Once unblocked, the mind may experience an expansion of awareness; a number of people have reported to me new levels of perception and communication after having these points treated.

As mentioned previously, it is desirable to focus upon the Throat center when trying to tap into the dream realm. Doing so allows one's thoughts to quiet down, enabling the deeper reaches of the mind to surface. This center appears to be the embodiment of the mystical "Open Sesame" that reveals the hidden inner dimension of the core. Normally, the development of this center naturally occurs as a person matures with age, if understanding and compassion have been previously established.

Brow Center

The Brow center in Sanskrit is called ajna, which literally means command, suggesting its dominant role in directing consciousness. The Brow center forms the active Yang pole along the psychoenergetic core. In Taoist phi-

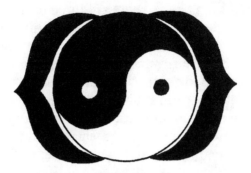

4-6 Brow Image

losophy, this is the Upper Field of Influence, linked to the heavens. In the Indian tradition, this is the upper Knot. Intuitively the Brow center is lodged near the center of the cranium, behind the eyes and within the brain.

The Brow center resonates most closely with the mind or mental sphere. Through this center's influence, the mind is able to identify with the past, present and future according to its karmic and biological preconditioning. Thus the mind is instilled with the awareness of time, for the purpose of organizing itself. On a cosmic scale, time and space are the primal duality that form the basis for the emergence of all phenomena. Time can be viewed as a creative potential, while space is its receptive counterpart. Furthermore, time and space are interpenetrating and coessential to each other's existence just like Yin and Yang. The Chinese images of heaven and earth are emblems for humanity's relationship to time and space, respectively.

Yet time is not without duality. Time is both illusionary, being bound to the transitory nature of human perception, and it is also real, since we cannot escape the progression of physical laws. Next I would like to discuss time, a difficult subject with many modes.

Within human beings there are three primary modes of time awareness: biological, subjective and archetypal. Biological or instinctual time appears to function as a physiological mechanism for regulating, harmonizing and protecting the body, especially the various organs, hormones and temperature, as well as the parts of the nervous system such as those linked with sensory and kinesthetic awareness. Biological time may have its physical moorings in the pineal gland, which is centrally located in the head. This gland is extremely light-sensitive and produces melatonin, a hormone that is crucial to the regulation of the body's natural rhythms. These rhythms (more accurately named circadian rhythms) become easily disturbed due to the deprivation of natural sunlight or by rapid long-distance travel. These rhythms are at times affected by cosmic influences, such as the moon, planets, sun and so on. If the body is unable to adapt to these subtle influences, its health is undermined.

In regard to subjective time, early human beings first began to consciously measure time in the paleolithic age, according to historians. This process of measuring time established a sense of order within the mind, and has been said to be an initiating factor in the establishment of civilization, distinguishing humanity from the animal kingdom. Unlike biological time, subjective time awareness does not suffer from long distance travel, since we can easily retain our memory of the sequential order of events. Memory is a vital component of what we call being conscious.

Curiously, modern human beings in general do not have a great sense of their own internal physiology and its distinctive biological rhythms. Apparently, we have moved away from biological time awareness and therefore from our instinctual self. It was Aristotle (384 - 322 BC) who said that since man has more reasoning power then beasts, he has fewer instincts.

I believe this movement of humanity away from nature and our instincts has left us dependent upon systems of healing based upon reasoning. In earlier times when humanity lived closer to the earth, it was the role of the healer or shaman to bring the sick individual back into accord with nature, through the shaman's use of his or her own instinctual knowledge. In these societies, the instinctual self was honored and cultivated as an important means to align one's self and others to life's rhythms and inner well being. Nowadays, many of the mental and physical problems human beings develop are a result of this loss of connection with nature's rhythms.

In our lives, subjective time orients awareness to the sequential movement of events perceived as past, present or future. Humanity's rational ability seems to be developmentally linked to a framework of time based upon an imaginary clock. Time has always been measured by man in the form of some type of rhythm: from pendulum clocks to modern oscillating quartz watches, to the regular waxing and waning of the moon. Early man seemed to first visualize a circular pattern to time, as in the lunar calendar or in the awareness of seasonal cycles derived from observation. This was followed later by a more linear model, which developed with the invention of numbers and mathematics. Jung has defined numbers as an archetype of order that has become conscious; thus, through time awareness we have a relationship to reality which has order and reason. Numbers appear to be the basic element of awareness of external order in the self-as-separate rational aspect of mind, and this can also link directly with our subjective sense of time. Yet subjective time can vary according to the individual, society and ethnic group. For example, two people will have different perceptions of the same week; for one person it may have gone by really fast while for the other it was tediously long. In my experience, disturbances in our biological time result in somatic disorders, while alterations in our awareness of subjective time lead to mental disorders.

The deeper the journey is made into the infraconscious level, the less subjective time and biological time exist. The time mode in the deeper recesses of the infraconscious (especially in the transpersonal) is called archetypal time, which is a more diffused quality of time. Archetypal time incorporates the notion of synchronicity and the interpenetrating relationship of time with space from a transpersonal level of truth. This form of time awareness is not limited by either biological or subjective time awareness. In archetypal time awareness there is a sense of "nowness," a fullness of the present that has both profound import and a "timeless" quality to it.

All three modes of time are, in experience, less distinct since they overlap each other, just as mind and body are inseparable in human life. Beyond this level of time awareness is the mystical state of no-time, where the duality of space-time is transcended.

While time awareness helps to shape and organize the mind, time consciousness and the mind are in the end an "illusionary" construction. Clearly, the mind does not exist by itself, since the mind is also a phenomenon being perceived. What is it inside of us that observes and responds to our own thoughts? The spirit is the seer; the mind belongs to the seen. In the Brow center, duality still exists as long as the self-as-separate oriented mind believes itself to be the source of consciousness and thus operates within the scope of subjective time awareness. Yet it is through the Brow center that the awareness of time can deepen into the archetypal mode that leads to the edges of no-time consciousness.

Normally, a center's vibrational frequency is denoted by its number of "petals." However, the Brow center has only two petals, representative of the primal duality of consciousness. Within the psyche, polarization occurs in various forms. For example, in each person there exists, psychologically, a tendency towards either extroversion or introversion, a leaning towards sanity or insanity, and physically, the differentiation of the brain into right and left hemispheres.

Functionally, the mind is composed of such conscious faculties as knowing, reasoning, rationalization, sensation, discrimination, intuition and integrative abilities. Apart from these available conscious faculties, there are the infraconscious realms. The mental sphere or mind oscillates within a polarized field between the conscious and infraconscious according to existing inner karmic patterns, all the time searching for stability and reconciliation as effective order. Proper functioning with orderliness is a primary aspect of the purpose of "mind".

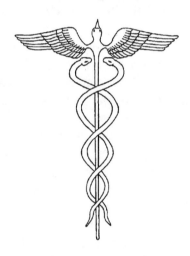

4-7 Caduceus

In its Greco-Roman form the staff carried by Hermes is representative of the axis mundi up and down which the journey between heaven and earth is made and primal duality overcome. The messenger gods of the Egyptian and Phoenician mythologies (i.e., Anubis and Baal) also carry similar wands. The caduceus was adopted by the medieval alchemists and physicians as a symbol of transformation and healing.

In Tantra this primal polarization within the mind is represented by the feminine-lunar (ida) and masculine-solar (pingala) channels. These subtle channels are thought to originate and separate from the Brow center, descending laterally and inferiorly along the psychoenergetic core. Essentially, the five centers below the Brow are visualized as energetic vortices or mandalas that arise from the approximation of the lunar and solar channels with the core, the dynamic points of overlap of the two energy channels. This is a marvelous image of primal duality becoming manifest.

The above archetypal image is wonderfully similar to the Caduceus, which in classical Greek mythology is the staff carried by Hermes (Mercury), the messenger of the gods. The Caduceus is composed of a central rod around which two serpents ascend and intertwine five times before their heads touch the wings of higher energy (i.e., the Brow center).

The Brow center's resonance with the mental sphere is the counterpart to the Vitality center's close association with the gross body. In each level duality emerges in its various forms. The natural place of reconciliation and harmonization of duality, in all its forms, is in the Heart center.

Through the Brow center the faculty of clairvoyance (the ability to see subtle energies and beings, past lives and even future events) can naturally develop. Clairvoyance is a distinctive feature linked to the archetypal time awareness state. This evolved faculty is noted in the realized mystic, shaman and sage.

A spiritual awakening within the Brow center is said to open the mystical third eye, allowing the experience of divine light to emerge. As Christ says in the gospel of Matthew: "If thine eye be single, thy whole body shall be full of light." This divine light is the pure essence of primordial energy, the source of all creation where no duality exists. The sage Zuang Zi says: "Pour into it and it never fills, dip into it and it never runs dry; yet it knows not a source; this is called the precious Light."

Psychologically, releasing the contents of this center brings forth an acceptance of oneself, others and life. During this time, relevant aspects of the transpersonal infraconscious become gradually illuminated and integrated. In the Brow center we find the seeds from which true wisdom emerges. Blockages in the Brow center are rooted in the inability to reconcile dualistic modes of thinking, negative attitudes and beliefs that are in opposition to one's ability to experience joy, love and compassion.

Crown center

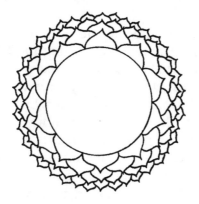

4-8 Crown Image

The Crown center in Sanskrit is called sahasrara, meaning thousand petalled, denoting the infinite vibrancy of cosmic consciousness. The Crown center is the passive Yang pole along the psychoenergetic core. This center is intimately linked to the transcendental-causal sphere which embraces the transpersonal infraconscious. There a creative capacity or potential resides, which the Taoists refer to as a Void. I believe this refers to a state of undifferentiated consciousness or a mode we do not ordinarily understand. I also believe this center acts as a bridge to this supraconscious state. Intuitively, the Crown center can be perceived as residing at the top of the head.

In India, the Crown center is called the Gate of Brahma, the creator. The Crown center is classically represented by a pure untouchable lotus plant that arises from the muddied waters below, which implies that this center is beyond the effects of the centers below. In Chinese theory the top of the head is referred to as a place were innumerable energetic pathways merge, which expresses the image of a powerful focal point, and parallels the Hindu idea. It also implies a unified state - all "paths" come from the Tao and lead back to the Tao, the single source.

I believe the Crown center helps to hold the spirit into its physical form, thereby supporting the Base center. A latent potential also exists within this center, a potential that is only activated when the spirit enters or leaves the physical body during the transitions of birth and death, or when one enters the state of samadhi, the divine union. The center's aroused potential can often be physically felt, as I have felt on others, as a distinct (but subtle) vibration on a newborn's fontanel or during the time of death, and for hours after the breath has departed, while the spirit departs. The heavenly gate of the Crown center is the preferred passageway for the spirit to depart the body, although any orifice is possible. Yet no matter which route the spirit leaves through, the Crown center will manifest this subtle activity while the potential is being activated.

The Brow and Crown centers represent complementary stages of mystic realization. The Brow center, the seat of the mystical eye, is where divine light is first seen. In this light the object of one's worship or a divine image may appear. But, ultimately these images do arise through one's own mind, originating from deep beliefs or religious impressions. Normally, a Christian does not have visions of the Buddha, for example.

The mystics say that these divine threshold images are paradoxical, functioning at first as vehicles and then later as obstacles to achieving final union. In the transcendent stage all awareness and identity with space-time are said to dissolve into cosmic consciousness. All duality is surrendered and wholeness is enjoyed.

The Seven Centers and Their Attributes

Base

- earth element
- square
- four petals
- passive Yin pole
- stores kundalini and past life memories
- grounds the spirit
- engenders the survival instinct
- seat of primal bonding

Vitality

- water element
- crescent moon
- six petals
- active Yin pole
- physical sphere's operative center
- engenders identification with the body
- reconciles the male-female duality
- seat of sexual identity

Solar

- fire element
- triangle
- eight petals
- absorbs and assimilates subtle energies
- opens into the personal infraconscious
- facilitates the emotions
- engenders the transformative ability
- seat of personal power and knowledge

Heart

- air element
- six pointed star
- twelve petals
- neutral pivot of the core
- engenders a harmonizing influence
- facilitates the integration of the infraconscious
- energetic sphere's operative center
- linked to dream realm and silver cord
- seat of love and compassion

Throat

- ether element
- circle
- sixteen petals
- facilitates communication and clairaudience
- allows access to inner realm
- engenders ability to articulate feelings
- seat of creativity and expression

Brow

- two petals
- active Yang pole
- mental sphere's operative center
- engenders awareness of time
- generates duality within mind
- facilitates the transpersonal infraconscious
- facilitates clairvoyance
- seat of wisdom and acceptance

Crown

- thousand petals
- passive Yang pole
- allows access to transcendental realms
- stores latent potential
- activated during birth and death
- linked to cosmic consciousness
- seat of the divine

Exercise 4
Imaging the Seven Centers

In Indian philosophy, the seven centers of the psychoenergetic core embody archetypal elements. We can use these metaphors to understand each center's role and nature, in both a general and a personal manner. In this visualization, I will give verbal clues to reflect on. Allow an inner unfolding of images and impressions to occur. In this way you can expand your awareness of the centers and help integrate their hidden aspects.

Start by finding a comfortable and quiet place to sit or lie down. This exercise will take about 20 minutes to complete. Uncross your arms and legs; close your eyes. Make a note of any intrusive mental thoughts, emotional feelings or physical sensations within your present awareness. Take a few deep breaths and with every exhalation imagine that you are breathing out these intrusive impressions. With every inhalation allow a feeling of peace and contentment to bathe your whole being.

The following words are designed to help you create an image of each of the seven centers. Read each center's description slowly. At the same time, permit your awareness to stay within the corresponding area of the body associated with a center. I will let you know the appropriate area to focus upon. Take a couple of minutes to reflect upon the center that you have just read before you move on to the next center. Let us begin.

The Base center is located in the perineum and is linked to the earth element. Reflect upon the image of earth. Imagine soil and rocks; earth's nature is solidity, it allows life to become embodied. Memories are buried and slowly a form appears.

The Vitality center is found in the pelvis and is associated with the water element. Imagine oceans and rivers; water's nature is fluidity; it allows life to flourish. Water is a generative force, from where all life emerges. Elusive inner tides and currents silently shift our beings.

The Solar center resides in the upper abdomen and manifests the fire element. Imagine fire and volcanoes; fire's nature is alterability; it permits life to change. Fire is the transformative capacity. Thoughts, energy and matter constantly change and reconstruct themselves.

The Heart center is located in the chest and is linked to the air element. Imagine winds and the breath; air's nature is mobility; it gives life movement. Vital energies circulate, day and night, within us all.

The Throat center is found in the neck and manifests the ether element. Imagine clear blue daylight sky; ether's nature is actuality; it allows consciousness to manifest. Our boundless nature reaches out and communicates with creation.

The Brow center is found in the head and is associated with time. Imagine the darkened night sky traveled by stars, planets, and moon; time engenders duality; it gives individuality. Through time, understanding and reflection emerge.

The Crown center is found at the top of the head. For a moment, imagine the possibility of an experience that transcends time, space, and elements. Allow a blissful unity and perfect contentment to reveal itself.

Slowly let your awareness return to your breath. Open your eyes. Take a few moments to reflect upon any images, thoughts or feelings that may have appeared. This exercise can be repeated in the above sequence or you can choose to focus on one or more centers during a session.

Chapter Five

The Embryonic Vessels

"Nature does nothing without a purpose." - Aristotle

I have always been fascinated by the orderliness of nature. Human beings come in a multitude of shapes, sizes, and distinctive features. Yet, there is also a profound common identity that allows us to relate to the humanness of each person we encounter. Within all of humanity's diverse races there is a basic and orderly development in the body's organization. Out of this arises a fundamental set of constitutional patterns that we all embody, to one degree or another. The underlying nature of this patterning is germane to our discussion about energy.

In the previous chapters, I have described the psychoenergetic core as having the primary function of orienting consciousness within the physical body and of organizing, through its vibrational resonance, the energetic terrain. In my understanding, the whole energetic system arises from and is continually organized by the psychoenergetic core. Essentially, the core embraces the mental and causal spheres where deeply held karmic patterns are found.

Commencing with this chapter, the focus will shift away from the psychoenergetic core to the other structures within the energetic terrain. First, a general outline of the energetic systems will be presented, followed by a detailed description of the embryonic vessels, which organize the development of the human body.

The Energetic System Outlined

Within the emerging human embryo, the psychoenergetic core is the initiating impulse from which all other energetic systems emerge. The psychoenergetic core first generates two energy fields in tandem: the embryonic vessels and the transverse currents. Both of these energetic phenomena are next in subtlety to the inner core.

Both the embryonic vessels and transverse currents are essential to the development, ongoing harmonization, and vitality of the physical, energetic, and mental spheres. Yet in comparison, the embryonic vessels are more closely associated with the body, while the transverse currents are closely linked to the mind. These currents wrap around the body, reflecting and impressing the vibrational quality and mental patterns of the psychoenergetic core upon the tissues.

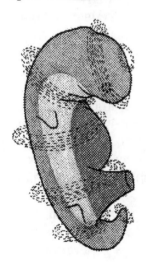

The embryonic vessels and transverse currents simultaneously manifest together during the first few weeks after conception, in the nascent tissues of the embryo. They form a complementary pair within the energetic terrain.

5-1 Embryo's Currents and Vessels

An artistic representation of the areas of influence and manifestation of the seven Transverse Currents and three Embryonic Vessels within the emerging human embryo.

Collectively, the psychoenergetic core, embryonic vessels, and transverse currents are structures that remain active throughout life. They are energetic potentials and organizing forces underlying the physical body's existence and mind's manifestation.

Furthermore, within the energetic terrain there are three distinctive physical or somatic systems: the cranial, visceral, and thoracic, which arise from the embryonic vessels and transverse currents. Each of these three systems expresses a unique energy pattern and physiological rhythm that allows the physical body to function properly and in harmony.

In addition, there is a subtle network of meridians in which energy, or Qi, flows. The meridians circulate along the surface of the body. These lines of energy are vibrationally dense, almost at the point of achieving material form. They are intimately connected with the interior of the body and to the three somatic systems. The meridians are the energetic terrain's exterior branches. They connect and help balance the energies within the cranial, visceral, and thoracic systems, and to a far lesser degree the embryonic and transverse currents. The meridians and the three somatic rhythms will be explored in greater depth in Chapters 9 and 10.

I have been fortunate to learn from many different methods in the healing arts and from different teachers over the years. The more I studied the more I found that energy and healing are viewed in amazingly similar ways throughout the earth. In particular, the embryonic vessels are an important concept that bridges many diverse ideas. Let us begin our journey outside the psychoenergetic core with consideration of these vessels.

Ancient Study of Anatomy

In formulating the concepts of the embryonic vessels and transverse currents, I owe my inspiration to the Chinese doctrine of the eight extraordinary vessels (ba mai). This ancient doctrine offers a sublime understanding of how human bodies develop within the womb. Only recently have comparisons been made between this theory and what we currently know about human embryology.

Amongst the Asian societies, the early Tibetans are noted for their great knowledge of human anatomy. Undoubtedly the ancient practice of celestial burial is the basis for much of their knowledge. In Tibet, this practice was and still is the most common method for disposing of a corpse. The undertaker cuts the corpse into small pieces which are then fed to vultures. Celestial burial arose from necessity, since firewood for cremation is limited on the Tibetan plateau and the earth is often frozen. This ritual practice is performed at special sites on high hilltops away from people's dwellings.

An impressive example of ancient embryological understanding is in the Tibetan text *The Four Tantras* (Gyu-zhi), written more than 1,100 years ago. This book describes the various stages of human embryological development, including human conception, the entry of the soul into the nascent embryo, and then the embryo's stages of growth through the aquatic, reptilian and mammalian stages. According to Tibetan Tantra, all the essential energetic and physical structures are manifest in the embryo by the eighth week in utero, which in modern science marks the end of the embryonic period.

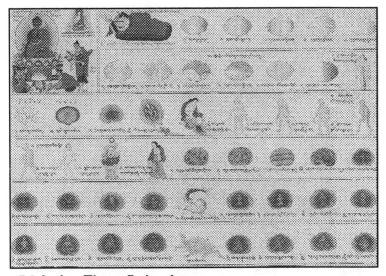

5-2 Ancient Tibetan Embryology

The above drawing is from the *Blue Beryl*, treatise of Sangye Gyamtso (1653-1705 A.D.), a compilation of 77 medical paintings that serve as a visual counterpart to *The Four Tantras* (Gyuzhi) an important Tibetan medical text of great antiquity. This painting depicts the normal development of the human form from conception to birth, including their physical, energetic and spiritual aspects. The various images show a rich material knowledge (such as cell division and stages of embryo-fetal growth) combined with great spiritual insights of subtler transformations.

The ancient Chinese were also quite aware of anatomy. They performed dissections on human cadavers and apparently did research on embryos. However, this early research was abandoned due to changing moral restraints, especially after the Han dynasty (which ended 220 AD), thereby leaving their studies incomplete. The Chinese did, however, borrow anatomical and embryological information from the Tibetans and Indians to complement their own knowledge. These early studies, supplemented by the meditative insight of the Taoists, led among other things to the development of the extraordinary vessel doctrine.

Extraordinary Vessels

According to Taoism and Chinese medicine, there exist eight subtle vessels which facilitate embryological development and supervise the physical and energetic structuring of the body. Also, they are thought to perform a life long role as energetic reservoirs, from which energy can be drawn during times of need. The extraordinary vessels are considered a distinct system apart from, but connected to, the surface meridians in which Qi flows. The eight vessels are functionally and structurally sub-divided into three groups: the primary, secondary, and belt vessels.

The primary vessels consist of the conception (ren mai), governing (du mai) and penetrating (chong mai) vessels. Embryologically, these three vessels are considered antecedent to the other vessels and are principally responsible for organizing the embryo's growth. The primary vessels are considered the most important of all vessels because they are thought to store the body's inherited Yin and Yang potentials.

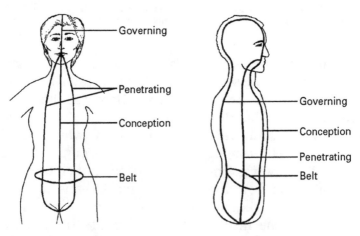

5-3 Primary Vessels

The three primary vessels (conception, penetrating and governing) run from the anus and genitals to the mouth in a longitudinal direction. Also shown is the belt vessel with its transverse trajectory around the waist below the navel.

Traditionally, the secondary vessels are composed of four bilateral routes that connect the four extremities with the head and trunk. They are called the heel (qiao mai) and linking (wei mai) vessels, both having a Yin and Yang division. Their function is to oversee the growth and organization of the limbs and meridians.

The secondary vessels are perceived to originate out of the primary vessels and are viewed as their external expression. Furthermore, the primary and secondary vessels have a complementary relationship: the inner primary vessels provide outward growth of the embryo, while the outer secondary vessels restrain this expansionary force. Thus, the secondary vessels function to protect and counterbalance the outward movement of the three inner vessels.

According to Taoism, the heel and linking vessels are associated with the lower and upper extremities, respectively. In fact, these vessels are often called the foot and hand vessels in Taoism. The Chinese character for heel (qiao) carries the image of heels lifting up while the character linking (wei) reflects the idea of hands pulling down. Therefore palms of the hands and soles of the feet are associated, respectively, to the Yin linking and Yin heel vessels; while the

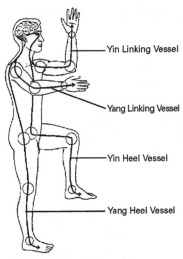

5-4 Secondary Vessels

The four secondary vessels connect the four extremities with the head and trunk. They run along the inside and outside of the arms and legs and are said to govern the twelve joints (i.e., shoulder, elbows, wrists, hips, knees and ankles).

backside of the hands and feet are identified with the Yang linking and Yang heel, respectively.

The belt vessel (dai mai) is the only vessel to have a transverse trajectory circulating around the waist below the navel, which is opposite to the other vessels in directional flow. Traditionally, there are two different viewpoints on the belt vessel. In traditional Chinese medicine, the belt vessel is an ambiguous structure unlike any of the other extraordinary vessels; its principal function is to harmonize the energy difference between the upper and lower body. On the other hand, the Taoists believe the belt vessel has multiple routes which extend in segments, from the head to the perineum. The Taoists perceive the belt vessel as a unique and distinct phenomenon that relates more to the psyche and the body's outer defensive barrier.

The belt vessel and the three primary vessels all originate from the vital gate, which is perceived to be located in the lower abdomen. In Chinese thought, the vital gate is considered the central hub of the physical and energetic spheres. I believe the vital gate is in fact the Vitality center of the psychoenergetic core. More will be said about this later in this chapter.

The Vessels Redefined

I have come to believe, from my research and experience, that these three types of vessels are for all essential purposes distinctive entities. Therefore, to distinguish my model from the traditional Chinese view I have renamed the vessels accordingly.

The primary vessels have been termed the *embryonic vessels*, to signify their key role in embryogenesis. Originally these vessels form outlines or energetic spaces within the embryo from which emerges the physical body's makeup.

The Chinese belt vessel corresponds in part to what I call the *transverse currents* which is a complementary, yet distinct, system. Light will be thrown on this in the next chapter.

In my opinion, the secondary vessels have only a supportive role in the context of the whole energetic terrain. In the Chinese model, the secondary vessels are used chiefly to explain the development of the limbs and meridian system in the embryo. I have termed these vessels the *peripheral channels* due to their sphere of influence. They are not a principal structure like either the embryonic vessels or transverse currents.

From a physical perspective, the peripheral channels correspond to various nervous system functions, especially within the brain stem (midbrain, medulla oblongata and pons). The brain stem governs the motor control of the body and is closely linked to the kinesthetic awareness of bodily movement and spacial orientation, as well as the regulation of the body's rhythms, including sleep. Interestingly, the brain stem is the first of the brain vesicles to develop in the embryo prior to the appearance of the limb buds, thus affirming the Chinese association of the secondary vessels with the head.

Compared to each other, the peripheral channels associated with the upper and lower extremities form a functional polarity. This is practically manifest by the opposite rotation of the limbs during their embryological growth and development. Looking from the

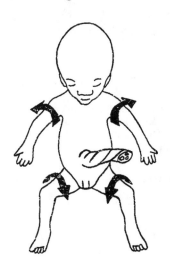

5-5 Limb Rotation in Utero

front, the lower limbs rotate medially around the long axis while the upper extremities rotate laterally.

The Embryo

In order to properly understand the three embryonic vessels, a study of the first few weeks of the embryo's life is crucial. This is the time when the physical body's structure and constitution will be determined. On the most fundamental level, human development begins from a single egg cell. Once fertilized, this single cell will generate an incredible series of events, out of which the embryo emerges.

Cells are the basic unit through which life can express itself. Cells are usually invisible to the naked eye. Within the human body there are about 350 different types of cells: blood, immune, lymph, nerve, skin, fat, liver, and so

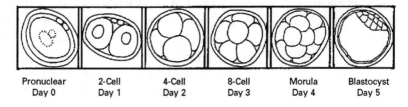

| Pronuclear
Day 0 | 2-Cell
Day 1 | 4-Cell
Day 2 | 8-Cell
Day 3 | Morula
Day 4 | Blastocyst
Day 5 |

5-6 a Initial Stages of Development
After conception cell division occurs in stages as shown in the above drawing. by day four the 32 cell zygote called morula (Latin for mulberry, for its shape) has descended through the fallopian tube. from out of the morula the blastocyst hatches and begins to adhere onto the lining of the uterus.

on. Cells have four intrinsic activities: they can multiply, change function, move in location and shape, and communicate with other cells.

The first two weeks following fertilization of the single-celled egg are marked by a rapid chain of cell multiplication and lateral expansion from which emerges a simple and disc-like embryo called the blastocyst. During the first two weeks all the cells appear and act in a rather similar fashion, as if their chief mandate is to multiply and implant onto the uterine lining.

5-6 b Blastocyst

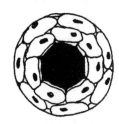

The implanted blastocyst on the uterine lining forms an amniotic cavity around day eight. Following this event some of the cells within the blastocyst flatten out to make a germ disc that is composed initially of two layers (of ectoderm and endoderm cells) followed by a third (mesoderm) layer forming in between them. A rudimentary placenta starts to manifest at this time to nurture the blastocyst.

© John Upledger, DO, North Atlantic / U.I. Enterprises, 1996

In the third week, the dramatic appearance of a primal pattern emerges. In embryology this initial patterning of the embryo's cells is called gastrulation. Essentially, gastrulation is the process that occurs when the cells of the blastocyst are rearranging and molding themselves into something that approaches the form out of which the human body will emerge. Thus, during gastrulation the body plan is laid down, including the body's spacial orientation into front and back, top and bottom.

The third week is the turning point in the development of the embryo. The cells are organized and readied for the metamorphosis of the coming weeks, for it is only after gastrulation that the organs, limbs, head, and brain will begin to develop. By the eighth week the cells within the embryo will have differentiated and matured themselves into what is essentially a miniature body or fetus. The metamorphic time from the fourth to the eighth week is referred to as the embryonic period. The remaining months of the fetus's time within the womb will be spent gaining mass, refining its physical features, and activating its various physiological functions.

During gastrulation the cells begin to move, contract, adhere, and generally mold themselves into an essential pattern. The cells align themselves into groupings from which they will springboard towards new areas, functions and divisions. Once this strategic plan is laid down, any deviation or damage to the cells will result in some sort of visible change to that being's future structure; prior to gastrulation the cells can easily nullify the consequence of any damaged cells.

Primary Tissue Layers

During the gastrulation phase, the embryo's cells align themselves into three primary tissue layers, called the endoderm, ectoderm, and mesoderm. This principal pattern of tissue layers is of great energetic and physical importance; these three layers are the origin of all the distinctive systems and tissues that will eventually become visible within the physical body.

By the beginning of the fourth week the embryo basically consists of three parallel axes: the rudimentary gut of mainly endoderm origin, the notochord of mesoderm, and the neural tube of ectoderm origins, from the interior to the exterior. This threefold pattern of the embryo's cells

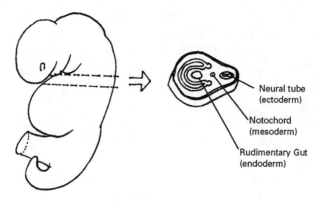

5-7 Embryo's Threefold Pattern

During the third week of embryonic growth the endo, meso and ecto derm tissues organize themselves to form the rudimentary gut, notochord and neural tube, respectively aligned from anterior to posterior.

will remain evident for about a week before rapid differentiation, specialization and movement occurs.

The eventual outcomes of the three distinctive tissue layers are as follows:

- *Endoderm gut* will go to form the abdominal organs related to the digestive tract, including the stomach, intestines, liver, pancreas and the respiratory tract;

- *Ectoderm neural* tube develops into the nervous system, including the brain, spinal cord and nerves, as well as the skin;

- *Mesoderm notochord*, being most diverse, produces the connective tissue, muscles, bones, bone marrow, blood and lymph vessels, spleen, heart, kidneys and gonads.

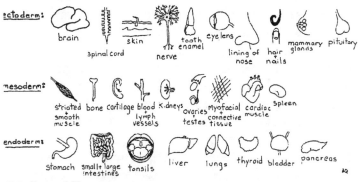

5-8 Fate of Tissues

The three primary tissues are the precursors for the various organs and tissues of the body that will eventually manifest. This illustration shows some of their eventual outcomes. © John Upledger, DO, North Atlantic / U.I. Enterprises, 1996

Dermal Tissues and the Embryonic Vessels

I believe the embryonic vessels form the energetic field or space for the manifestation and development of the three dermal tissue layers. I have named the three vessels according to their initial embryological positions. The Anterior vessel stimulates the formation of the endodermal rudimentary gut; the Middle vessel forms the mesodermal notochord; the Posterior vessel develops the ectodermal neural tube.

Using the Chinese terminology for the vessels, the conception, penetrating and governing vessels respectively correspond to the Anterior, Middle and Posterior embryonic vessels. In Chinese medical theory, the conception vessel is called the ocean of Yin; its route rises up the body's abdominal midline. The governing vessel is known as the ocean of Yang, having a route that moves up the spine. The external routes of both the conception and governing vessel start in the anus and terminate in the mouth. The penetrating vessel is traditionally called the ocean of the twelve meridians, organs, and of both the Yin and Yang aspects. This vessel is visualized as having a bilateral route situated between the conception and governing vessels.

Essentially the Anterior and Posterior vessels form a complementary pair, in which the embryologically more aggressive Yang neural tube enfolds the more passive Yin rudimentary gut. Furthermore, the above mentioned classical meeting places of these two vessels (i.e. the anus and mouth) correspond to the sites of ectodermal and endodermal fusion at both ends of the embryonic disc, while the Middle vessel creates the energetic space for the mesodermal layer which forms the notochord in the embryo. From the mesoderm all the body's bones, muscles and connective tissues are formed. The connective tissue or fascia plays an important energetic role, which is that of being the physical medium for the meridians. More will be said about this later. Thus, in terms of polarity, the Middle vessel is neutral. In terms of spatial relationship, the Middle vessel is between the two other vessels, just as the mesoderm is physically in between the endoderm and ectoderm.

The Primitive Node

Central to this whole process of embryonic differentiation of ectodermal, endodermal, and mesodermal tissue is the physical structure called the primitive node. The primitive node is crucially important because it acts as a hub for cell proliferation and organization. From an energetic perspective, the Yang ectoderm, being more active, initiates the separation between itself and the Yin endoderm. The resulting polarization generates a potential that manifests in the form of mesoderm.

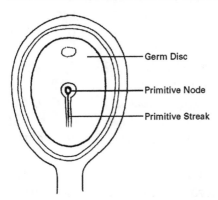

Germ Disc

Primitive Node

Primitive Streak

5-9 Primitive Node

The primitive node and to a lesser extent the primitive streak act as a hub for cell proliferation and organization within the embryonic germ disc. Via the node, the mesoderm layer arises in between the ectoderm and endoderm layers.

The primitive node, I believe, is the physical reflection of the Vitality center, the active Yin pole along the psychoenergetic core. The primitive streak appears to be the reflection of the Base center, the passive Yin pole. The physical form of both primitive node and streak does recede into insignificance; they are no longer clearly identifiable within the fetus. The embryonic vessels all arise from the drama at the node. These vessels then form spaces in which the bodily tissues are organized and purified energies are stored, acting somewhat akin to batteries.

In Chinese terms, the node is the physical manifestation of the vital gate. Metaphorically, the node is the seat of a void, the Taoist term for the precursor of all material manifestation and structure.

Extended information for the technical reader on the keynote embryonic process is given in the attached box. The general reader may prefer to omit this part, at this point.

Keynote Processes in Embryonic Development

What follows is a brief description of the various tissue changes that occur immediately before and after the appearance of the primitive node.

After the blastocyst has implanted itself into the uterine wall and a rudimentary placenta is established to give support, some of the blastocyst cells flatten out to form a disc. Initially this embryonic disc is composed of two distinct layers of endoderm and ectoderm cells, then a third layer of mesoderm cells forms in between them. This three layered disc extends out from the blastocyst's wall into a cavity. The part of the disc that remains attached to the wall will become the tail end of the embryo, while the part that protrudes into that cavity will become the head of the embryo. [See Illustration # 5-10.a]

Gastrulation, the first major event of the third week, commences with the appearance of a faint midline structure, the primitive streak, within the ectoderm layer near the inferior or tail end of the bilaminar germ disc [See Illustration # 5-10.b]. At the superior end, the primitive

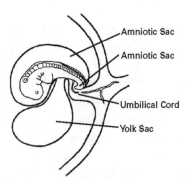

Amniotic Sac

Amniotic Sac

Umbilical Cord

Yolk Sac

5-10.a Orientation of Embryo

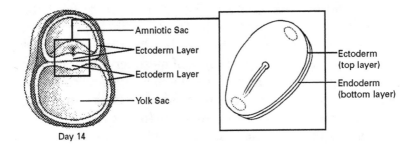

Day 14

5-10.b Bilaminar Germ Disc

streak swells to form a knot or node. Ectodermal cells migrate towards the primitive streak and node; once they are there, invagination occurs, forming a linear furrow or groove in the primitive streak and a pit in the node [See Illustration # 5-10.c]. These migrating cells move in

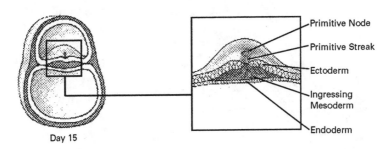

Day 15

5-10.c Trilaminar Germ Disc

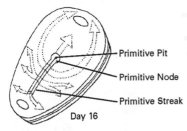

Day 16

5-10.d Primitive Streak and Node

Dotted lines and arrows represent paths of migration of ingressing mesoderm that arise from the epiblast (primitive ectoderm) cells.

between the ectoderm and endoderm to produce an intermediary mesoderm layer. [See Illustration # 5-10.d]

Thus, during the first few days of the third week the embryo resembles a bean seed with a superior pole, a hilum and an inferior pole. The primitive node is at the level of the hilum; inferior to the node is the primitive streak and superior is the prechordal plate. The prechordal plate is a compact mass of mesoderm tissues that prevent the proliferating intermediary mesoderm from extending too far superior. All these structures run along the midline of the embryo. At both the extreme inferior and superior ends the endoderm and ectoderm remain fused. The conjoined superior end later develops into the oral and nasal membranes of the head, while the inferior end gives rise to the perineum and lower orifices of the pelvis. [See Illustration # 5-10.e]

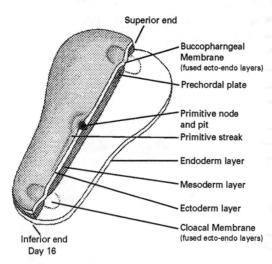

Superior end

Buccopharngeal Membrane
(fused ecto-endo layers)

Prechordal plate

Primitive node and pit

Primitive streak

Endoderm layer

Mesoderm layer

Ectoderm layer

Cloacal Membrane
(fused ecto-endo layers)

Inferior end
Day 16

5-10.e Embryo as Hilum

Rapid proliferation of cells occurs from the primitive node and to a lesser degree from the primitive streak. Out of the primitive node a hollow tubular column of mesodermal cells grows superiorly along the midline axis towards the prochordal plate to form what is called the notochord. [See Illustration # 5-10.f] The notochord is the structure around which the future vertebral column will develop; it also serves to induce the formation of the nervous system from the overlying ectoderm. Lateral to the notochord, mesodermic tissues differentiate into three

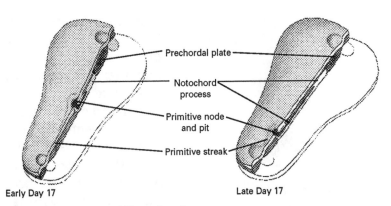

Early Day 17   Late Day 17

5-10. f Appearance of Notochord

sections: paraxial, middle and lateral. The three mesoderm sections will eventually differentiate into the following: out of the paraxial mesoderm arises the axial skeleton, voluntary musculature and parts of the dermis of the
skin; from the middle mesoderm the kidneys, adrenals
and gonads are produced; and from the lateral mesoderm
the fascial linings of the organs, body wall, musculature
and sub-dermis develop in due course. [See Illustration #
5-10.g] Meanwhile in the region of the primitive streak a

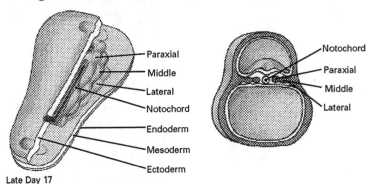

Late Day 17

5-10. g Notochord and Mesoderm Sections

small passageway, the neurenteric canal, forms, creating
a brief temporary connection up between the ectodermal
and endodermal layers. [See Illustration # 5-10.h]

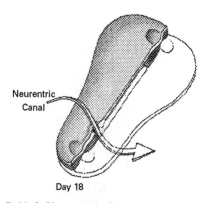

Neurentric Canal

Day 18

5-10. h Neurentric Canal

The canal allows for communication between ecto and endo derm layers, as well as, between yolk and amniotic sacs.

As soon as the paraxial mesoderm cells manifest they develop into a series of rounded, whorl-like structures called somitomeres. These somitomeres form into paired blocks on either side of the notochord and neural tube (see below) just beneath the ectoderm. The first pair of somitomeres appear in what will be the base of the skull and continue to grow in an inferior direction towards the tail. A few of the somitomeres will disappear and the remaining ones, called somites, will serve to segmentally organize the axial skeleton, including the vertebral column, parts of occipital bone in the base of the skull, voluntary musculature of the neck, trunk and limbs, as well as part of the dermis of the neck and trunk. [See Illustration # 5-10.i]

The nervous system itself originates from the ectoderm situated over the notochord. During the third week the ectoderm layer thickens into a plate and then invaginates along the midline-axis to form the neural groove. [See Illustration # 5-10.j]

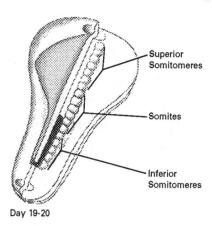

Superior Somitomeres

Somites

Inferior Somitomeres

Day 19-20

5-10. i Somitomeres and Somites

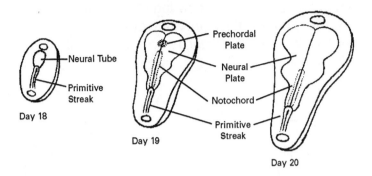

Day 18

Neural Tube

Primitive Streak

Day 19

Prechordal Plate

Neural Plate

Notochord

Primitive Streak

Day 20

5-10. j Neural Plate Development

The elevated lateral edges of the neural plate form into folds; as the neural groove deepens, the lateral folds begin to approximate. By the end of the third week they fuse into the neural tube. This fusion commences in the region of the future neck and spreads in a longitudinal direction. The primitive streak which originally extended half the developing embryo's length progressively becomes an anatomically insignificant structure in the sacral-coccyx region by the end of the embryonic period. [See Illustration # 5-10.k]

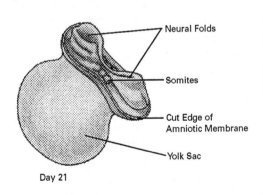

Neural Folds

Somites

Cut Edge of Amniotic Membrane

Yolk Sac

Day 21

5-10. k Neuralization

Another important structure, the rudimentary (or primitive) gut, is formed towards the end of the third week by the enfolding of the embryonic disc. Because the developing neural tube grows more rapidly from the peripheral area, this results in longitudinal and, later on, transverse folding of the embryonic disc, making it a more cylindrical, bean-shaped design, as mentioned previously. [See Illustration # 5-10.l]

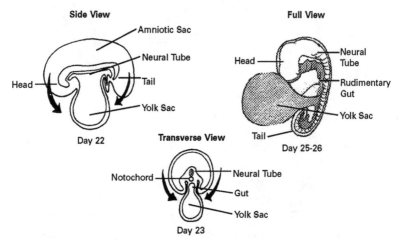

Side View
- Amniotic Sac
- Neural Tube
- Head
- Tail
- Yolk Sac

Day 22

Transverse View
- Notochord
- Neural Tube
- Gut
- Yolk Sac

Day 23

Full View
- Head
- Neural Tube
- Rudimentary Gut
- Yolk Sac
- Tail

Day 25-26

5-10. l Rudimentary Gut

All of the above mentioned cell migrations occur within about 10 to 11 days, a rather short period of time.

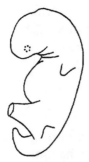

5-10. m Appearance of Limb Buds

The upper limb buds first appear around day 24 while the lower limb buds around day 28.

Immediately after the cells have repositioned themselves into the three layers of gut, notochord and neural tube, a metamorphosis begins within the embryo. During the fourth week the growing heart will begin to beat, the buds of primitive organs will appear, and the head and brain start to distinguish themselves. This is followed by the appearance of the limb buds towards the end of the fourth week. [See Illustration # 5-10.m]

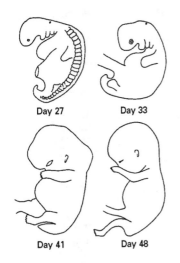

Day 27   Day 33

Day 41   Day 48

5-10. n Developmental Series

The human embryo grows in leaps and bounds from the forth to the eighth week. The following are the approximate normal lengths for the above figures in utero: day 27 - 5mm, day 33 - 10mm, day 41 - 15mm and on day 48 - 20mm (at this point the embryo weighs about 2 grams).

From this point, a steady development occurs in the embryo. By the eighth week, the embryo is fully developed, possessing all human characteristics, and hereafter is called a fetus. [See Illustration # 5-10.n]

The Embryonic Vessels and Their Resonance

As a unit the embryonic vessels are closely aligned to the physical body, giving it both its form and constitutional traits. Individually, each vessel engenders its own tissue and organizes the body in a unique way. Furthermore, each of the embryonic vessels helps in the establishment of an inherent somatic system that generates a physiological motion within a specific locale. The three distinctive somatic systems and their motions will be discussed in Chapter 8. As well, the three embryonic vessels are closely linked with the Chinese concepts of essence, Qi and spirit.

The important linkages between the vessels and specific areas and tissues are outlined in the following table:

	Anterior	**Middle**	**Posterior**
Polarity	Yin	neutral	Yang
Dermal Tissue	endo	meso	ecto
Initial Form	primitive gut	notochord	neural tube
Main Body Site	abdomen	chest	head
Principle Tissues	visceral	musculoskeletal	nervous
Somatic System	visceral	thorax	cranial
Somatic Motion	visceral motility	breath & heart beat	cranial rhythm
Substance	essence	Qi	spirit

Biological Constitutions

In used to determine the biological constitution of an individual, because of their preeminent role in initiating and structurally patterning the physical body. Biological traits have been associated with the concept of the three dermal tissues in western literature since Dr. W. H. Sheldon's landmark discovery of the mind-body connection to the dermal layers in the 1940's. But, a much older and enduring body of knowledge from the east, that of Ayurveda, has also given us a wealth of knowledge based upon the human constitutions. I believe the constitutional types that Ayurveda proposes, without perhaps saying so, are also based upon the same biological patterning level. This is no wonder, because the three dermal tissues are the most fundamental building blocks of the physical body.

For his part, Dr. Sheldon proposed that a person's physique predisposes that individual to certain behavioral temperaments. His interest was in the mind and the emotions. He accepted that consciousness not only influences the physical body, as we can see in so many psychosomatic disorders, but also that the physical body can and does influence consciousness. He sought to bridge these two views.

According to Sheldon the three embryonic tissue types form a primary and important basis for understanding an individual's physical makeup and mental disposition. He systematically classified the physical body's characteristics into three groups: endomorph, ectomorph and mesomorph, based upon the three tissues. He found that each of these three body types generates its own associated behavioral patterns which he called temperaments. The three temperaments according to Sheldon can be summarized as follows:

Endomorph:
physique- predominance of fat; the visceral organs
are proportionally more spacious;
the body is soft and round.
temperament- relaxed; sociable; loves to eat; love
of bodily comforts; affectionate.

Ectomorph:
physique- fragile; a sensitive and developed nervous system, with large cranium; delicate skin;
slender and tall frame.
temperament- sensitive; restrained and inhibited;
tends to worry and is often fearful;
artistic; likes solitude.

Mesomorph:
physique- bones, muscle and connective tissue are
well developed; a strong muscular frame,
as in an athletic build.
temperament- highly active; likes exercise;
assertive; courageous.

Sheldon did not see the temperaments as being rigid or exclusive. Rather he said individuals usually have an ascendancy of one type with varying degrees of secondary characteristics from the other types. His method gives a general picture, based on physical constitution of an individual's character type. It was not meant to replace in-depth psychological analysis. Sheldon's theory of temperaments was also incorporated by physical medicine to assess and classify natural variations of human physique.

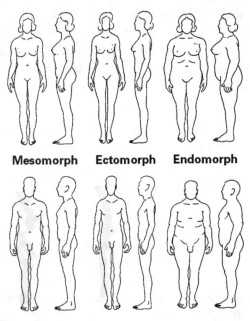

Mesomorph   **Ectomorph**   **Endomorph**

5-11 Body Types

This representation shows the three male and female body types that are based upon Sheldon's theory of temperaments. This illustration is taken from a standard text on orthopedic physical assessment.

The ancient science of Ayurveda, from a totally different paradigm, holds similar views about the physical body's effect upon consciousness. The Ayurvedic system is of course much more complete. As such, this system of biological constitutions or temperaments includes a greater in-depth survey of the possible character traits, including physique, appetite, taste preference, emotional and mental tendency, pulse, speech, sleep, skin complexion, and so forth.

As explained in the tri-dosha theory of Ayurveda, in each of us there are three tendencies, called doshas, which are condensations of the basic archetypal elements within nature. Every person will manifest varying levels of dosha activity according to their unique inheritance. As well, the doshas are used to describe both normal and pathological variances. This differs from Sheldon's temperament theory, which relates mostly to non-pathological tendencies. However, for the most part Sheldon's temperaments do correspond with the doshas of Ayurveda. Dr. R. H. Singh, in *The Science and Philosophy of Indian Medicine,* affirms this view. Specifically, the endomorphic, ectomorphic and mesomorphic temperaments corresponds to kapha, vata and pitta doshas of Ayurveda, respectively.

Below, in the chart, is a summary of the leading traits of the three doshas and human constitution:

Kapha: large, solid build, tendency towards obesity; good stamina with steady energy, but has tendency to underexert; regular appetite and steady sex drive; pale, oily skin, tans easily; enjoys temperature and seasonal changes; quiet, affectionate and calm disposition; learns and forgets slowly; tendency towards possessiveness; avoids confrontation; sleeps easily, rises with reluctance.

Vata: light, thin build, tendency towards being underweight; poor stamina, energy comes in bursts, with a tendency to overexert; variable appetite and sex drive; skin is dark and tans easily; prefers warmth; talkative; learns and forgets easily; often worries and is fearful; excitable, changing moods; light interrupted sleep.

Pitta: medium build; medium stamina, periods of intense energy, overexerts when competing; intense appetite and sex drive; skin often light and sunburns easily; prefers coolness; speaks with purpose; learns quickly, forgets slowly; tendency towards anger, irritable under stress; enterprising with a sharp intellect; sleeps and rises easily.

These Ayurvedic differentiations and characteristics are treated in greater detail in my book, *Tao & Dharma: Chinese Medicine and Ayurveda*, written with Dr. Robert Svoboda.

In my practice, I regularly use the concept of the three constitutional types of Ayurveda to assess my patients and to determine which treatments are most appropriate and how they will react to the different treatments I give them. By knowing their constitution, I can even modify a technique to best suit their nature. For example, I once had a decidedly Vata person, Carol, who came to see me for acupuncture. She was suffering from insomnia and stress. She appeared anxious and agitated. Carol worked in a high powered lawyer's office. She was thin and didn't care too much for routine or food in general. She lived a lifestyle that she couldn't keep up with, while her energy changed from day to day. She complained of terrible mood swings. By listening to her symptoms and story I knew that she was a Vata person. This was confirmed by reading her pulses and looking at her tongue. The pulses and tongue are the preeminent diagnostic tools of Ayurveda. Thus, by understanding Carol's constitution, I knew that when I used acupuncture I must modify this technique to her Vata nature. Carol had a predominance of mental energy that resulted in a finely tuned, highly sensitive nervous system. In this case, I had to avoid using too many needles, leaving them in too long, too deep or with too much stimulus. Only in this way would the best results be achieved and her symptoms diminished and doshas balanced.

I hope this brief introduction has served to articulate my belief that the embryo's three primary tissues and their eventual outcomes do engender the body's biological features or constitution. At the root of this constitutional patterning are the embryonic vessels. Throughout life the embryonic vessels profoundly affect the physical body and mind through the vital energy they store. The embryonic vessels are not static entities but undergo subtle and continual change just like a person's temperament. Through understanding the embryonic vessels and linking them to the human temperament, a profound therapeutic model can be created.

Exercise 5
Microcosmic Orbit Meditation

Based upon an ancient Taoist practice, this meditation engages all three of the embryonic vessels. You will be circulating energy around both the back and front of the head, chest and abdomen. This route follows the evolutionary path of the ectoderm and endoderm, which is respectively upwards toward the head and downwards to the abdomen. In addition you will be using the breath, governed by the mesoderm, to propel and balance the energies. Thus, the Anterior, Middle and Posterior vessels will all be engaged. The Taoists refer to this as harmonizing heaven and earth.

The Microcosmic Orbit Meditation is an excellent exercise for reintegrating the mind and body. I often suggest this meditation to people who perform vigorous spiritual or energetic practices; it helps counterbalance their side effects. I find that there arises a state of inner peace and a sense of wellness from performing this exercise.

First, position yourself in a chair with your back relatively straight and comfortable, feet flat on the floor and your arms resting on your thighs or the chair's armrests. Adjust your head so that it sits relaxed and comfortable. Close your eyes. Lightly place the tip of your tongue on the inside upper gums just above the teeth. Once you are relaxed and in position, sense how you are; notice any physical sensations, feelings or intrusive thoughts that may be present, then let them be.

Starting with your inhalation, imagine energy arising from your anus, then moving into the base of your spine, upwards along the spine through the back, neck and into your head; keep moving it over the inside and back of your head to your third eye (in between and behind the physical eyes). As you

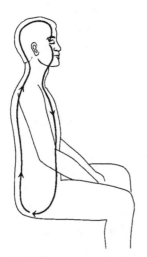

exhale, imagine energy going down the midline of the body from the third eye, let it descend through your face into your tongue, down the throat, sternum and along the front of the abdomen, all the way to the pubic bone along the pelvic floor to the

5-12 Microcosmic Orbit

anus from where it started. You have completed one orbit.

With each coming breath repeat this procedure, moving the energy up the back during inhalation and down the front during exhalation. Try to focus your awareness about an inch or so below the skin's surface and let your breath soften and deepen as you go on breathing; each time allow your breathing and imagery to merge into a nice rhythm. About 10-15 minutes is an adequate length of time to do this meditation.

After you have stopped the exercise, sense how you are. Notice any changes in your sensations, feelings or thoughts. Slowly move about and pay attention to how you feel over the next few hours.

CHAPTER SIX

The Transverse Currents

"If thine eye be single, thy whole body shall be full of light." - Christ

The distinction between the psychoenergetic core and transverse currents can best be illustrated using the allegory of the sun and its light. Sunlight is a separate, diffused emanation from the sun. They are separated by both time and space, yet sunlight is wholly dependent for its existence upon the sun. But, still, we cannot say that the light is the sun, only a manifestation of it.

Similarly, the currents are manifestations of the core operating (like sunlight) according to certain inherent laws or patterns. Nevertheless, one can feel the currents directly and infer the state of the core through them, just as we are able to perceive sunlight and infer many things about the sun from a distance. However, it should be said that just as our perception of the sun is altered by the earth's atmosphere, so the psychoenergetic core is obscured by the nature of mind and by the body through which the currents pass. The purpose of this chapter is to explore the transverse currents and their significance to the mind and body.

Together, the embryonic vessels and transverse currents operate as a complementary pair within the energetic terrain. The transverse currents are more Yang in polarity, resonating closely with the mental sphere. In contrast the embryonic vessels have more of a Yin quality, being linked to the physical body's development. The source of both the vessels and the currents is the psychoenergetic core, which harmonizes and stabilizes them.

Initially, the transverse currents arise out of the Vitality center within the psychoenergetic core, thereafter emanating as segments or rings from the crown of the head to the perineum of the pelvis. In early embryological growth, the primitive node is physically representative of the Vitality center. This node is the root of both the transverse currents and the embryonic vessels. The transverse currents assist in restraining the lateral expansionary force of the embryonic vessels. Furthermore, the transverse currents absorb excess energy from the embryonic vessels, thereby helping to regulate the overall potency of energy within the body.

Each separate transverse current is a field that operates in sympathy with one of the psychoenergetic centers (i.e. the Crown, Brow, Throat, Heart, Solar, Vitality and Base centers). Each current continually expresses a center's vibrational frequency upon the tissues within its orbit. However, the polar end currents are very compact, without a broad orbit. They serve to complement the restraining function of the two polar centers; otherwise they are of little consequence. Therefore, apart from the two polar currents there are in total five active transverse currents.

Another important function of the transverse currents is to facilitate the polarization of the tissues within the embryonic currents. This polarization process occurs after the embryo's third week. Essentially, the endoderm tissues within the Anterior vessel start to migrate, accumulate and differentiate in the lower portion of the embryo's trunk; the ectoderm tissues within the Posterior

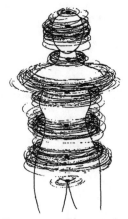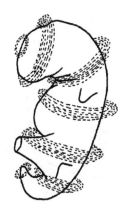

6-1 Transverse Currents in Adult and Fetus

Each transverse current is a field operating in sympathy with a psychoenergetic center. Within this system the top and bottom currents have a restaining function congruent with the nature of the Crown and Base centers while the five currents in between assume active roles. Viewed from above to below the seven psychoenergetic centers and their associated current are as follows: Crown - Top, Brow - Head, Throat - Neck, Heart - Chest, Solar - Abdomen, Vitality - Pelvic, and Base - Bottom. The figures show an artistic representation of the transverse currents in both a fetus and adult.

vessel undergo a like process in the opposite direction, towards the emerging head. Thus, the more Yang-like ectodermal nerves are focused within the head, becoming the brain; the more Yin-like endodermal gut goes on to form most of the abdominal tissues. This polarization is initiated and mediated by the transverse currents under the guidance of the psychoenergetic core.

For their part, the mesoderm tissues of the Middle vessel become diffused throughout the evolving embryo, although the physical heart (being mesoderm in origin) acts like a central hub for all the mesoderm. Thus in their eventual outcomes, the three tissues will change orientation from simple longitudinal lines within the embryo to a more horizontal alignment. The meaning of this will be further explored in Chapter 8.

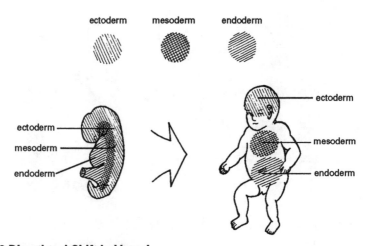

6-2 Directional Shift in Vessel

The transverse currents facilitate the reorientation of the embryo's tissues from an initial longitudinal axis to a more horizontal alignments.

The Five Currents

For all practical purposes, there are five active transverse currents, as there are five functionally active centers within the psychoenergetic core. The five active currents are linked to the psychoenergetic centers as follows: head current to Brow center; neck to Throat; chest to Heart: abdomen to Solar; and pelvis to Vitality.

Like the centers, each current has a different perceivable vibrational frequency, from higher to lower frequency in a descending order. Using the analogy of sound, the transverse currents are vibrating in tune, but on a lower octave, with the centers. Thus, the currents' effects are felt right down into the physical body. Ideally, each current's frequency harmonizes the physical tissues and energetic structures within its orbit of resonance. The psychosomatic application of this principle, of consciousness diffusing itself, will be addressed in the coming chapters.

The specific spheres of resonance or orbits of the five active currents can be described as follows:

Head – includes the whole of the head

Neck – between the base of the skull and the top of the shoulders (the thoracic inlet)

Chest – between the thoracic inlet and diaphragm

Abdomen – from the diaphragm to the crest of the pelvis

Pelvic – all of the pelvic area to the perineum

The most important routes, in general, are the Head and Pelvic currents, relating respectively to the Brow and Vitality centers. The Head and Pelvic currents set the tone and responsiveness of the whole system. The Head current is Yang in polarity and the Pelvic current is Yin. The Chest current also plays an important equalizing and integrating role within the system, just as the Heart center preforms this function within the core.

Furthermore, there is a transverse field generated down the extremities, as a natural extension of the main currents. We can think of these currents within the four limbs as operating in unison with the peripheral channels to regulate the extremities, on an energetic level. I envision the extremities to generate six primary and bilateral orbits around the main joints: shoulder, elbow and wrist in the upper limbs and the hips, knees and ankles of the lower limbs. These joints are important sites for the energetic regulation of the extremities.

The Aura

The transverse currents also have the important function of generating an energetic protective barrier for a person's body and psyche. This barrier appears outside the body's outer surface as a shell-like etheric field or aura.

Besides the emanations of the currents within the aura there are also filtrations of other energetic influences emanating from the meridians, organs, blood, nerves and other tissues, as well as the mind.

Overall, the size and integrity of the aura is primarily related to the transverse currents, and secondarily to the states of the various influences filtering into the aura. However, rapid changes can occur within the aura as a result of the secondary influences; for example, an emotional disturbance will immediately imprint itself into the aura. Usually, secondary influences that imprint upon the aura are transitory in appearance, unless they become chronic in origin. A degree of "fixation" is what chronic means.

Extending beyond the aura, which primarily expresses the vibrational frequencies within the physical and energetic spheres, there may be other subtler layers of the aura reflecting refined aspects of mind and spirit. The question of how many layers exist as distinct from the etheric aura is a subject of controversy amongst the various commentators on this phenomenon. For example, B. Brennan, in her book *Hands of Light*, ascribes seven layers to the aura, while the eminent C. W. Leadbeater refers to four layers in his book *Man Visible and Invisible.* Indeed, a person's belief system may actually engender these differences in what is perceived within the aura. No two people perceive reality in the same way, as we realize when we consider that a work of art will elicit a unique and personal interpretation when viewed, based on the viewer's experience, understanding, and disposition. This includes acquired tastes, both intrinsic and conditioned by education and other influences or required values.

Indeed, I have always been fascinated by how we human beings perceive the world around us. Take vision, for example. The eye can discern more than a million colors and can respond to a single quantum of light (which is the smallest amount possible). Some of us have incredible visual acuity, while others have much less. Then there are individuals, blind from birth, who have developed an acute sense of hearing or some other faculty as a compensation for the loss of sight. All of us have differing perceptual abilities, whether visual, auditory, kinesthetic or otherwise. Just as certain people have an ability to hear a wider range of sound, some individuals are able to visually perceive a subtle dimension that most people do not notice. This ability may be learned or may be a natural gift. This subtle dimension that is perceived is composed of many energetic patterns with complex wave forms and resonances. For those with sensitive vision, the etheric aura is the distinguishing feature that stands out around the human body, as in all living things.

To see auras, a person needs to have an open mind and relaxed disposition, as well as a certain amount of mental clarity. Children and unsophisticated people have a natural ease in perceiving the aura. In a healthy person the etheric aura is compact, emanating between 2 - 10 centimeters from the skin surface, and appears as a silvery white hue. Changes to the compactness as well as coloration of the aura all indicate imbalance of one sort or another. In modern science, Kirlian photography (developed in Russia during the 1950's) has allowed the aura to be captured on film. Kirlian photography is now used in some eastern European hospitals to assess medical problems or to anticipate their development. [See Illustration # 6-3]

Furthermore, apart from the subtle hues or colors that manifest within the aura, the human body also projects electromagnetic radiation in the form of infrared heat into this same field. This infrared heat is not uniformly projected off the skin; there are natural variations in temper-

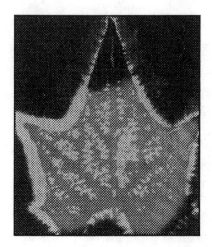

6-3 Kirlian Photograph

All living forms have auras including plants, animals and human beings. This kirlian photograph shows a leaf and its energy field. Note that the top of the leaf has been cut off, yet the aura still remains whole. This "phantom leaf" phenomenon occurs only if the remaining plant is large and vital enough to withstand loss of its physical integrity. Perhaps this energetic phenomenon explains why many human amputees retain awareness of their missing limbs.

ature depending upon such factors as metabolic rate, menstrual cycle, digestive activity, disease activity and so on. In my experience, the aura proper tries to contain the infrared heat within its field. Thus for practical purposes they are the same. In practical terms the aura is an important energetic structure that ties in with the body's immune system and thermal regulation. In addition, both the aura and infrared heat can be utilized in diagnosis to determine disease. Unfortunately, the scope of this book does not allow for a detailed analysis of the aura.

Certain natural expansionary or visionary drugs such as peyote or ayahuasca can also facilitate the perception of auras. Indigenous people in the Americas have used these medicines for sacred inner journeying and shamanic healing purposes for countless millennia. One area of my personal research has been with the tradition of ayahuasca, a drink that is made from the combined synergy of the bark of a jungle vine (banisteriopsis caapi) and the leaves of a different plant (psychotria viridis). Ayahuasca is a sacred Quechua word meaning the vine of the soul, commonly referred to as yage.

Ayahuasca is used to enter the visionary state, in which the drinker journeys into the deep realms of the psyche, into the personal and transpersonal infraconscious. Some call this realm the crystal sphere, because of the luminous visions and the alteration of space-time awareness that occurs. The Indian rishis would rightly tell us that all that appears within this realm reached via expansionary drugs should be recognized as a manifestation of one's own consciousness. Most fascinating is that the rituals, prayers and experiences of the Amazonian ayahuascaqueros (those who imbibe the magic drink) bear remarkable resemblance to the description of the worshipers of soma, the psychotropic drink of the ancient Vedic culture of India.

A common practice amongst indigenous people in the Amazon is in the ritual use of head feathers, which they say reflects their awareness and honoring of the aura. Practically, this knowledge or awareness is believed to have been inspired through the use of ayahuasca and other visionary substances. In fact, most traditional cultures throughout the Americas ritually use smoke to smudge and feathers to purify a person's aura.

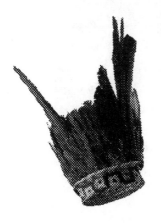

6-4 Head Feathers

These head feathers come from the Brazilian Amazon region where indigenous people have long used sacred plants to gain deeper insights into life. Head feathers are expressions of the hidden beauty and power that exists within our subtle body and its aura.

I have also found the utilization of the transverse flows of energy in the Peruvian ritual called karpay, a healing ceremony that dates far back into pre-Incan times. According to Dr. Jose Cabanillas, an expert on the cultural medicines of Peru, during the karpay the healer respectfully asks that the Apus (spirits of the mountains) send down good wind (i.e., energy) that is able to work with Pachamama (mother earth) to heal the patient. As well, the healer uses coca leaves, water, fire and other elements of nature during the healing ceremony. During one part, the healer moves stones in a circular direction around the periphery of the patient's body, being careful not to make physical contact between the stone and the body. The circles are performed in various places that approximate the positions of the transverse currents. The use of stones is said to help cleanse and balance the person's energy.

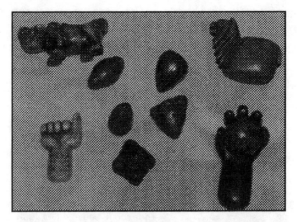

6-5 Incan Sacred Stone Artifacts

The above sacred objects, called *cuyas*, are used for healing and spiritual purposes. In rituals they are usually held in the hand by the healer-priest and applied either over or directly onto the body (in the form of acupressure) to balance the subtle forces within the body.

I have found that most indigenous cultures use the invocation of deities or sacred teachers to empower spiritual or healing energies upon a person or group. These energies are brought into the healing through gift-waves (or specific streams of energy) as directed by the healer. For example, the Tibetans call upon the Medicine Buddha Vaidurya before preforming a medical procedure. In South America certain jungle tribes chant Icaros, the sacred name or sound of a plant, which can help draw a particular plant deity to oneself for healing purposes; the Christians use prayer for the invocation of divine grace.

Transverse Currents and Their Sphere of Resonance

Let us return to the transverse currents proper. As I have already mentioned, each transverse current transmits, at a lowered octave, the vibrational frequency of a single center within the psychoenergetic core. As a result, all the physical tissues and structures within a current's orbit will tend to resonate together, so that the endocrine glands, nervous tissues, organs, and so on, all function in sympathy and harmony.

Physically, the natural variations of mechanical pressure within the body's head and trunk are illustrative of this idea of energy differentiation along orbits or planes outlined by the transverse currents. Naturally, the internal pressure differences originate from the pulmonary system, while laterally oriented structures (i.e. diaphragm, thoracic inlet, etc.) within the body act to withstand, redistribute and harmonize the varying pressures. The reported normal values of these pressures are:

skull +15 cm H_2O

neck +5 cm to +10 cm H_2O

chest -5 cm H_2O

upper to mid abdomen +5 cm to +20 cm H_2O

lower abdomen to pelvis +20 cm to +30 cm H_2O

In regards to the pressure variances, the transitional areas between the transverse currents play an important role. These sites also have similar physical features; specifically, they house an unusual abundance of laterally oriented fascial tissue (i.e. the craniocervical juncture, the thoracic inlet, the diaphragm, perineum and to a lesser extent the pelvic arch). The lateral structures function to regulate pressure variations and prevent disease processes within the mind or body from spreading out of a current's sphere. Yet, under certain circumstances these same structures may also become key places where energy restrictions occur. More will be said in the next chapter about this in relation to the meridians and the fascia.

Similarly, in Indian and Tibetan medicine and Yoga, the subtle Prana (equivalent to the Chinese concept of Qi) is differentiated into five types according to their directional movement and to their pertaining transverse segment of the body. These bear a relationship to the above mentioned pressure changes linked to the transverse currents. Specifically, within the sphere of the Pelvic current in which the "downward-moving air" (apana) operates and is said to manifest; the "equalizing air" (samana) is found within the Abdomen current. The "forward-moving air" (prana) which absorbs the breath's life force is centered within the Chest current. The "upward-moving air" (upana) circulates within both the Head and Neck currents, while the "pervasive air" (vyana) circulates around the body like the etheric aura and is centered in the heart.

It should, however, be noted that these so called "airs" have many more functions than just moving energy in certain directions.

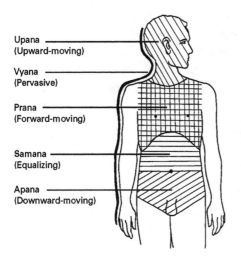

Upana
(Upward-moving)

Vyana
(Pervasive)

Prana
(Forward-moving)

Samana
(Equalizing)

Apana
(Downward-moving)

6-6 Five Forms of Prana

This figure shows the five essential forms of Prana which bear striking resemblance to the concept of the transverse currents. According to the ancient classics, when Prana's five subtle forms operate with a healthy potency and within their respective spaces a person remains balanced, if not illness is likely to occur.

Glands, Nerves and the Five Currents

By studying the endocrine glands and nervous system, we can also find clear relationships amongst the transverse currents. Many of these relationships are only now being understood, and they promise to be of great clinical value. For the purposes of discussion, the following is a summary of major endocrine and nerve correspondences with the transverse currents:

Current	*Endocrine Gland*	*Nerve Plexus*
Head	pituitary-pineal	brain stem-cranial nerves
Neck	thyroid	brain stem-cervical
Chest	thymus	cardiac
Abdomen	adrenal-pancreas	celiac
Pelvic	gonads	hypogastric-sacral

Changes within a current will directly impact upon the mental and energetic spheres, and vice versa. For example, the Head and Pelvic currents resonate with the brain stem and sacral segment of the parasympathetic nervous system, which functions to induce a relaxation response important to proper digestion, mental calmness, sleep, sexual arousal, and so on. These two functional ends of the transverse current system are the key areas for regulating and setting its tone, and for influencing the body's self-healing potential.

The body's four largest sympathetic nerve plexuses - cervical, cardiac, celiac and hypogastric - appear within the orbits of the Neck, Chest, Abdominal and Pelvic currents respectively. The sympathetic nerves have an excitatory effect upon the body's tissues, organs, glands and muscles. They have an opposing action to the parasympathetic nerves. The sympathetic system triggers the fight or flight response, a natural response in stress.

The major endocrine glands also point to a five-fold division of the body that corresponds to this transverse current model. These endocrine glands physically manifest the refracted patterns of the psychoenergetic core via the transverse currents. For example, the conscious awareness of time associated with the Brow center has its physical manifestation in the pineal gland, through the hormone melatonin. And the urge to unify the inner male-female duality,

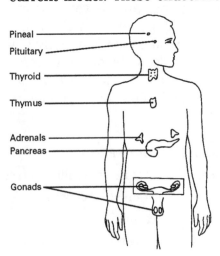

Pineal
Pituitary
Thyroid
Thymus
Adrenals
Pancreas
Gonads

6-7 Endocrine Glands

governed by the Vitality center, is physically in sympathy with the ovaries and testes and their secretions. The others, too, have their psychic relationship to the deeper levels. However, I would not directly connect these glands, nerves or other tissues to the psychoenergetic centers; rather, the intermediary mechanism of the transverse currents is responsible for these resonances.

Mind, Emotions and the Transverse Currents

In relationship to the mind, the transverse currents function to diffuse and orient consciousness throughout the physical body. Each current organizes a particular aspect of consciousness, which is in congruence with its corresponding psychoenergetic center. Furthermore, mental patterns and emotions (such as fear, grief, anger, worry and so on) tend to stay within their associated current's sphere. For example, grief associated with the Chest current is connected to the Heart center because this is the seat of love, grief being a natural expression of love's loss.

This entrapment of a feeling or thought within a current is a natural protective mechanism preventing the person's mind and body from becoming overwhelmed. The psychoenergetic core and transverse currents facilitate the ordering of consciousness in this way. However, when an emotion or thought is suppressed or habitually maintained, it can become pathologically anchored within the physical tissues of a current. When these pathological emotions and thoughts leave their normal entrapment and wander into adjunctive currents the greater will be the tendency towards disorder within consciousness.

Furthermore, the physical body tends to store feelings and thoughts primarily in fascial tissues. Fascia is a form of connective tissue that lines structures like the muscles, tendons, bones and organs. Once anchoring of feelings and thoughts occurs, there is a general reduction in the overall capacity for feeling and clear thinking by the individual, including the somatic tendency for tension in the fascia and musculature. This tension can be both pervasive and tenacious, producing a guarded state. This state of somatic guarding further assists the individual in coping with whatever emotional stimulus there may be. However, this form of coping does not lead to resolution or healing; in fact it often becomes a contributing aspect in the maintenance of the imbalance.

The following is a list of basic feelings which in my experience can be linked to the transverse currents.

Current	Feeling
Head	pride, self doubt, neurosis
Neck	loneliness, emotional withdrawal, hysteria
Chest	jealousy, grief, shame, possessiveness
Abdomen	anger, worry, greed, indecisiveness
Pelvic	fear, insecurity, powerlessness, lust

Of course, because no two human beings are alike, the above list of feelings is only a rough guide. The transverse currents are an important energetic structure that facilitates the melding and communication between the mind and body. Influencing the currents will generate positive changes in both the mind and emotions.

Fundamentally, the transverse currents and the etheric aura that they project are extremely important for the integration and protection of the mind and body. Diagnostically, we can learn to use the aura to sense the currents. For example, once I had a patient, John, come to me for extreme nerve pain in his back and down his sciatic nerve in his left leg. John had been in a motorcycle accident in which he injured himself. His pain was intolerable after the crash; he was operated upon and his lower back fused. Following the operation his pain was still there, but it was more or less bearable. He searched from practitioner to practitioner, from therapy to therapy, looking for relief. When I saw him, over a year had passed since his accident. I examined him and in doing so I assessed his aura and found that his Head current was in fact the most dysfunctional, more so than his Pelvic current where his complaint was situated. I found on closer examination a number of cranial restrictions deep inside his skull. I focused my attention upon the head and gave only secondary consideration to the lower back and leg. In a short time his condition improved and he started to live pain free. Although he had no pain in his head, this subtle cranial disturbance was part and parcel of his injury and it impeded the lower back's proper healing. It was by diagnosis of his aura that the primary trauma was properly located in the energetic terrain.

Exercise 6
Sensing the Aura

All living beings have an energy field that radiates outside the surface of their physical form. The etheric aura is a significant part of that energy field. In this exercise you will try to sense and influence the aura with your hands.

You may do this exercise either standing or sitting. Whichever you choose, let yourself relax in that position, at the same time maintaining a relatively straight spine. This exercise can take between 10 - 20 minutes.

Begin by closing your eyes and noticing how you feel. Now, take a few deep breaths, and with each exhalation imagine that you are breathing out the stress and tension from your body. Then bring your hands together and start rubbing them. Concentrate on the sensations that arise from your hands as you gently rub them all over. Do this for about a minute. Then separate your hands out in front of your body so that the palms are facing each other. They should be about two feet apart from each other. Ever so slowly bring the palms toward each other, all the time monitoring with your hands the sensations that arise. As your palms get closer to each other, attempt to sense a field or barrier between your hands. There will be a distinct sensation when the aura of the left and right hands meet. This sensation is like experiencing the surface tension of water, such as when your flat hand meets the surface of a calm body of water. Play with this surface tension when you have discovered it. Slowly move your hands closer together and then further away. Do this a few times. Do you sense a resistance that seems to separate your hands as you approach the barrier? Is there a sense of the hands becoming attracted to each other after you have crossed the barrier?

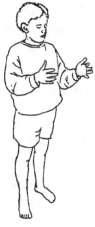

6-8 Sensing Aura

Once you have done the above steps, you can explore other parts of your aura or perhaps a partner's aura. In the beginning you may find it helpful to keep your eyes closed; this will help to focus your mind. But after some practice you can easily keep your eyes open when sensing the aura. Also, the presence of multi layered or synthetic clothing can sometimes affect the projection of the aura. Remember to begin by positioning your hands a couple of feet off the body and slowly moving them towards it. You can use both hands when you are working with a partner. It is better to keep your hands separated from each other as you sense the aura.

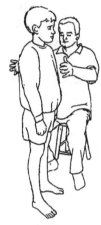

6-8 Sensing Aura with Partner

When you are working with a partner, try going over his or her whole aura. Start from the head and work down. Make a mental note of areas in which a difference is felt in the barrier's distance to the body's surface. In a balanced aura the aura's barrier tends to be relatively uniform. If the aura isn't uniform then this can be due to physical, energetic or mental restrictions manifesting in that part of the system. Sometimes rapid fluctuations do occur in a person's aura when he or she is experiencing an unusual or intense stress, whether mental, emotional or physical. This is normal. Proper and thorough analysis about the causes of what is showing up in the aura is always appropriate before jumping to any conclusions. Diagnosis is beyond the scope of this book. We shall focus attention on the existence of the aura and not its clinical significance.

After you have acquired a clear impression of the aura, you can add a further step, which is to differentiate temperature changes in the aura as you are scanning with your hands. For sensing temperature it is important not to linger too long (more than a couple of seconds) with your hands in any one place. This is important because heat exchange starts to occur when your hands remain stationary over the skin of the other person's body. Sensing temperature is best done in conjunction with a partner; it is difficult to sense heat variations on yourself. Curiously, research has shown that both deficiency and excessive disease conditions will be felt as heat by your hands. Thus, by this method we can not judge the nature of a condition but only its location.

CHAPTER SEVEN

The Meridians, Qi and Fascia

"One small needle cures a thousand illnesses." -
traditional Chinese saying

In the spring of 1982 I had the opportunity to study acupuncture in China. This was my first trip to Asia, a continent that I had been attracted to for years. The airplane landed in Hong Kong, and from there I proceeded by train across the border to Canton in communist China. At that time westerners were still a novelty in mainland China, which was only just beginning to emerge from its long period of isolation. At the Canton train station I found a People's Liberation Army display with a free clinic on traditional Chinese medicine and western medicine. Amongst all the people and activity, men and women were getting treated right there in front of everyone. They were receiving traditional massage, some were being given information on nutrition and the prevention of malaria, others were having acupuncture treatment or vaccinations, and yet others were being informed about birth control; these are just a few of the displays that I remember. Western and Chinese medicine were obviously working together side by side. Being the only foreigner around, I was given a gracious tour of the free clinic and was asked many questions. They were also delighted to hear that my purpose for being in China was to study their healing art of acupuncture.

The next day, I headed by train from Canton in the south to Beijing in the north where I was to study. En route, I started to get ill, starting with a fever, headache and burning sensation in the eyes. I had come down with conjunctivitis, an infection of viral or bacterial origin that affects the eyes. I felt very sick. My companion in the sleeping compartment was an elderly army officer who, upon noticing my condition, found an army doctor who was also on the train. I was given some western medication to help me through the long train trip. The drugs helped to temporarily ease my pain and to reduce the fever. When I arrived in Beijing, I was told by my school that I should at once start receiving acupuncture and Chinese herbal medicine for my conjunctivitis. Immediately after the first acupuncture treatment the fever subsided, and by the next morning my eyes started to clear up. In less then two days the illness had passed. They told me that Chinese medicine is the preferred method for the treatment of conjunctivitis.

With each passing day in my training, I became more and more impressed by the effectiveness of Chinese medicine and acupuncture. I remember one of my teachers, Dr. Liu, who was as distinguished and wise as he was old, and who had a remarkable ability to manipulate energy through the use of a single needle. Dr. Liu could generate a very real and perceptible hot or cold sensation that he could move around in your body. He would accomplish this by inserting an acupuncture needle in a meridian point on your body and then, through his mental intent, breathing and manipulation of the needle, he would direct the Qi as he wished. When he manipulated the needle he would gently twirl, thrust and move it sideways under the skin.

Every day I saw people coming to the hospital ward to receive treatment. In time most of these people got better.

They came with visual and hearing problems, headaches, hepatitis, depression, insomnia, gallstones, backache, sciatica, menstrual difficulty, thyroid deficiency, diabetes, epilepsy, asthma and a myriad of other complaints.

One typical case was that of a young man in his early twenties, Yao-ling, who was having increasingly frequent asthma attacks. He had been referred by the medical doctors to us for treatment since western medicine failed to control his symptoms. Every second day my clinical teacher, Dr. Yi, and I would use a combination of acupuncture and moxibustion to treat Yao-ling's condition. The young man was also given herbal medicine to supplement the acupuncture and moxibustion therapy. In a month's time Yao-ling was greatly improved, his attacks were now infrequent and his general breathing was much fuller. He also noted feeling more calm and inwardly balanced. Treatments were gradually reduced to once a week and then every two weeks as his health improved. Eventually treatments would be left to his discretion, whenever he felt the need for them.

There are many similar stories of other conditions. We treated infants just weeks old and elderly people brought in on stretchers. We treated chronic and acute illnesses alike. There was always a flow of people through the clinic, and usually we saw about sixty people each morning. Sometimes our therapy was not so successful, and those cases were referred for other forms of therapy, including western medicine. Our hospital was mainly focused on traditional Chinese medicine, having about a dozen different out-patient clinics which used various traditional approaches or specialties, such as massage, herbal medicine, Chinese pediatrics or gynecology. Some conditions, like acute bacterial infections that needed antibiotics or surgical cases, we never saw at all since these folks went directly to the western medicine departments of the hospital.

This is not a perfect world, and the Chinese health care system that I observed certainly had its deficiencies. However, I felt a lot of compassion and caring by the practitioners. I was deeply impressed by the healing effects of this ancient system that is based upon concepts of energy and the interconnectedness of life.

I believe that Chinese medicine's enduring legacy is due to its highly sophisticated art of acupuncture and the concept upon which it is founded: there exists a flow of Qi within a subtle system of meridians. In my experience these lines of energy are real and not imaginary. With training, we can directly perceive these meridians and learn to manipulate them when needed. Knowledge about the meridian Qi flow allows us to better understand the subtle links between the various parts of the body, the interrelationship of disease symptoms, and how the mind and emotions impact upon the tissues.

Here in the western world we are slowly embracing acupuncture and other forms of oriental medicine. While the public demand for the use of these systems grows by leaps and bounds, the medical community's acceptance of them lags far behind. In my own practice I see more and more people using my services for prevention and resolving problems before they become chronic, and this differs greatly from ten years ago when the greater majority of my patients came to me out of desperation, seeing acupuncture as a last resort when all else had failed. My practice of acupuncture has evolved through incorporating my own experience and knowledge while adapting the techniques and theories that I learned in China to the western culture and the individual constitutions of my patients. What follows are my thoughts on the nature of Qi, the meridians and the physical medium in which they operate.

Meridians and Qi

Chinese medicine recognizes there are different types of Qi, depending on their location and function. For example, there are defensive, nutritive, original, cosmic, organ and meridian forms of Qi within the human body. Qi can also inhabit, concentrate and become stored in certain tissues, such as bone marrow. In the case of the organs, Qi represents the functional capacity and physiological action of an organ. The concept of organ Qi is intimately related to the meridian system, since both organ Qi and meridian Qi communicate and flow into each other. In theory, meridian Qi also derives part of its vitality from the organs.

Unfortunately, Chinese physicians did not develop any comparable theory regarding the nervous system, which remained obscure until the advent of modern medicine. In Chinese medicine, the operations of the nervous system are included under the rubrics of various theories, especially of the spirit and, secondarily, the organs and meridians. In treating illness, traditional Chinese medicine perfected the use of meridian stimulation, which included the use of acupuncture, massage or moxibustion (mild cauterization using ignited herbs) upon specific points along a meridian's course.

According to Chinese theory, the meridians flow along the peripheral portion of the body under the surface of the skin, connecting internally with the organs. Meridians are subtle structures that have small openings or points along their passageways. Altogether there are over three hundred and fifty recognized points along the meridians. Each point has an array of functions that may be unique to itself or linked to the meridian in which it is found. I have written a book on this subject called *Acupuncture Points: Images & Functions*, which describes the meaning

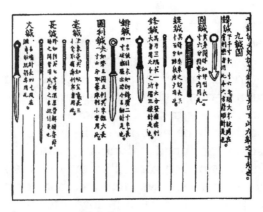

7-1 Ancient Acupuncture Needles

Since ancient times Chinese medicine employed a variety of needles made out of various common metals in the art of acupuncture. Some of the larger needles were used for bloodletting and skin scrapping, however these practices are not so popular today. Nowadays most acupuncture practitioners use fine stainless steel needles that are inserted without pain, although a number of mostly pleasant sensations can sometimes accompany the arrival of Qi at the site of the needle; these include warmth, tingling, heaviness, and a floating sensation for example.

of the acupuncture point names, their traditional functions and their modern medical indications.

While in China, I met researchers who were actively studying the meridian system. Their research involved needling specific acupuncture points on highly sensitive people who had no prior understanding of Qi or meridians. These patients reported subjective sensations during needling which corresponded closely to the meridians' routes. There was an approximately 85% rate of accuracy recorded between the subjective descriptions of the patients and the traditional descriptions of the meridian routes.

In comparison, modern research has had only limited success trying to link the Qi phenomenon with the nervous system. Rather the opposite seems to have emerged, i.e., that the meridians are an independent phenomenon. The pathways of the meridians do not necessarily follow nerve pathways, and meridians can be activated by acupuncture stimulation done on points with little nerve

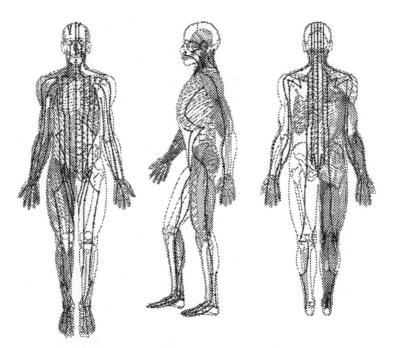

7-2 The Meridians

According to traditional Chinese medicine, the human body possess twelve bilateral and two unilateral meridians with a total of 670 acupuncture points that manifest along their routes. However, other energy channels and points have been described in Chinese medicine but generally they are of lesser clinical significance. The accompanying illustration depicts the external pathway of the fourteen major meridians. © Nielsen/Garbett, 1995

supply. Certainly, though, nerves and Qi do impact on each other, although they are separate phenomena.

Indeed, all living things possess Qi and possibly meridians. This has been well documented in animals. Less known is the fact that research in China has confirmed that plants can also possess meridians. I was told of this research during my first stay in Beijing by a guest lecturer who had studied the effects of acupuncture upon trees.

I perceive, in humans, the meridians as being subtle structures in nature. There does, however, appear to be a physical medium through which they operate. For intrinsic purposes the meridians use the body's fascial system as their conduit. The emerging meridians in the embryo develop with the appearance of the limb buds and primitive organs. The external routes of the meridians are organized under the guidance of the peripheral channels, as mentioned before. The whole meridian network traditionally is thought to mature gradually, accompanying a child's physical growth and becoming fully developed by puberty.

The Fascia

The fascia has certain characteristics that make it an ideal physical medium for the circulation of Qi, especially in the form of meridian Qi. Fascia is composed primarily of collagenous and elastic fibers within a colloidal or glue-like ground substance. Collagen fibers are highly pliable and tough, and form the bulk of the fascia, while elastic fibers are stretchable, giving fascia greater flexibility. The majority of fascial fibers in the body orient themselves in a longitudinal direction. Although the fascia is a continuous network, three types of fascia are differentiated: superficial, deep, and visceral.

Superficial fascia lies beneath the skin, covering the whole body with variations in thickness. This layer functions principally to maintain body heat, store fat, and help protect the body against trauma. Superficial fascia is thinner in males than females. Deep fascia molds into the body walls and extremities. It covers and holds muscles, tendons and ligaments together, as well as separating them into functional units. Deep fascia allows for free muscle movement, covers the blood and lymphatic vessels, and surrounds the bones, brain and spinal cord. Deep fascia does not store fat and is more dense than superficial fascia. Visceral fascia, which is also known as subserous fascia, envelops and supports the internal organs; it lines the body cavities in the form of pleura and

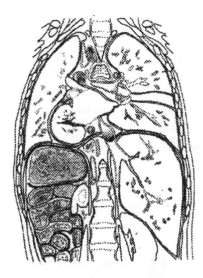

7-3 Fascia of the Body's Trunk
The fascial sheaths and layers of the various organs, muscles, bones, etc. of the abdomen and thorax are penned in as the darker lines. The three types of fascia (superficial, deep, and visceral) are interconnected and meld together to provide an ideal physical medium for the circulation of Qi.

peritoneum. Visceral fascia anchors various organs to stabilize them structurally.

Fascia, from a functional and structural perspective, is a single, continuous, mobile sheet of connective tissue wrapping itself around virtually every structure inside the body. Fascia allows for an amazing amount of responsiveness because of its mobility and elasticity. Via the fascia, pain, tension, and stress are easily diffused and rapidly communicated throughout the whole body.

According to my clinical investigation, the classical routes associated with the meridian system utilize and follow the body's fascia. Specifically, the superficial fascia corresponds to the meridians's exterior pathways and the deep and visceral fascial layers to its internal pathways. In this way, the meridians are able to communicate with the organs, nervous system, and interior structures of the body. Specifically, visceral fascia helps the meridians to directly communicate with the organs, while the deep fascia helps the meridians connect with the brain and spinal cord.

Indeed, all the fascial linings act as energetic envelopes which protect and maintain any particular structure's integrity. For example, I have found acupuncture influences the organs, bones, and musculature directly when needle stimulation is given to a structure's lining (respectively, the visceral fascia, periosteum, and myofascia). Furthermore, there is a discernable but slight differentiation of energetic quality in each type of lining.

Qi and the Fascia

As the conduit for meridian Qi, fascia is distributed throughout the body, enabling it to facilitate communication within the body. Furthermore, fascia is highly responsive to electrical and magnetic influences. Fascia under the guidance of Qi is a sensitive biological amplifier of subtle external forces. Changes of season, temperature, weather, atmospheric pressure in the biosphere and the various influences of the sun, moon, and planets in the celestial sphere all have an impact upon the physical body through the meridian Qi. The various levels of fascia allow the meridians to communicate with virtually any part of the body. The fascia aids the meridian Qi to protect the body and in regulating temperature.

In healthy tissue the colloidal ground substance of fascia provides a semi-fluid medium for the passage of immune system cells. The fascia has limited blood and nerve supply. Generally fascia is also aligned longitudinally, like the meridians. However, there are important lateral planes as well. Often these lateral planes are located between the transverse currents. The base of the skull, the thoracic inlet, the respiratory diaphragm, the pelvic diaphragm and to a lesser extent the top of the pelvis are all examples of lateral structures where fascia is abundant. Each of these structures is found in between or along the periphery of a transverse current.

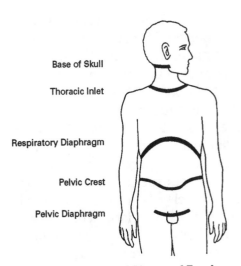

Base of Skull

Thoracic Inlet

Respiratory Diaphragm

Pelvic Crest

Pelvic Diaphragm

7-4 Important Lateral Planes of Fascia

Generally, an imbalance within a transverse current tends to cause meridian Qi and other subtle energies to become blocked. This blockage often arises along the laterally oriented fascia and musculature. Physically, the laterally aligned fascial tissue is an important component for absorbing, harmonizing and re-transmitting variations of internal pressure.

Of all the lateral fascial planes, the respiratory diaphragm is probably the most significant. The diaphragm has a central role in the reciprocal relationship between breath, Qi and mind. For example, when the normal flow of Qi is disturbed by one's thoughts or emotions, immediate changes to the breath will occur. Breath is said to vitalize both the Qi and the blood. Abnormal breathing patterns, in turn, affect the vitalization of the Qi, creating a vicious cycle. Energetically, the diaphragm is often the site of powerful suppressed emotions and physical tension. No wonder so many disciplines incorporate breathing techniques to release energy and for spiritual transformation.

In treating patients, I frequently use gentle hands-on manipulation to release the various transverse fascial fields. When I am treating the respiratory diaphragm, patients often feel an emotional and physical release as the energy unblocks. This is followed by an immediately noticeable softening of the patients' breath.

A Brazilian colleague of mine, Dr. Francisco de Souza, has related a highly illustrative clinical story about the connection of fascia and meridian Qi. He performed acupuncture needling to one patient's kidney meridian using a point on the inner ankle. Almost immediately an indented groove manifested itself along the kidney meridian from the site of the needle to the groin of the patient, where the kidney meridian enters the trunk of the body. The superficial fascia became clearly taut exactly along the classical description of the meridian. When I was studying in China my teachers also described similar experiences with spontaneous meridian manifestations. Generally, these occurrences are rare, but they do confirm the findings of many practitioners who believe fascia is the primary medium of the meridians. In Dr. de Souza's case, he was fortunate enough to photograph this phenomenon, which I have reproduced here with his kind permission.

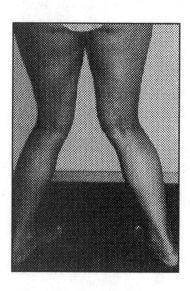

7-5 Meridian Qi Manifestation Photograph

This rare photograph of a spontaneous meridian manifestation shows an indented groove running along the insides of both legs following acupuncture needling. The tautness of the superficial fascia along the leg segment of the Kidney meridian allows for clear visibility of its course. According to Dr. de Souza, this seven month pregnant patient was being treated for a kidney infection which was accompanied by edema and low back pain. In her case the trunk portion of the Kidney meridian was less affected and visible.

Energy Vortices

In the previous chapter, the transverse currents were discussed in relationship to somatic guarding, while the fascia and musculature were identified as tissue sites where suppressed thoughts and feelings are stored. Often at these tissue sites an important phenomenon can manifest. I simply call it an energy vortex. Let me explain.

In modern society there are many manufactured chemicals, from mood-altering antidepressants to highly addictive drugs like cocaine, that radically alter normal awareness. In nature there are plants, from hallucinogenic mushrooms to cannabis, that are equally capable of altering awareness and loosening the cohesion of consciousness. Although poorly understood, the brain is able to produce its own potent chemicals that can alter the mind's perception and the body's health for better or worse. Usually, feelings or thoughts, and to a lesser extent dietary imbalance or physiological stress, initiate these internal chemical changes. Everyone has felt, at one time or another, the organic force that an emotion may produce. At times, charged emotions are uncontrollable, producing a fission-like reaction within consciousness and an equally strong physiological response.

Normally, the mind and body are able to process emotions with relative ease. When emotions become habitual or repressed, however, there is a far more complex dynamic present. At the center of habitual or suppressed emotions is a psychic process, a complex or configuration, that has become lodged within a specific site in the body as a charged energy vortex. Whenever a familiar thought, sensation or feeling arises which resonates with one of these repressed energy vortices, a physical and emotional reaction is generated that is usually explosive or implosive in nature.

Often, at the center of a psychic complex is an experience that is unrecognizable, intense and frightening to the conscious mind. These overwhelming experiences usually exist because the original traumatic event or emotion occurred when one's awareness was too immature to identify and integrate them, for example in early childhood. In later life when one contacts the center of a psychic complex, the experience is re-lived. This crisis offers the opportunity for that experience to be healed through consciously identifying and integrating into awareness the re-lived experience. However, to get to the center of a psychic complex there are usually many associated feelings and memories that require contact and re-integration and reduction of their energetic potency. Of course later life traumas and shocks can also generate similar complexes.

Energy vortices, depending upon their resonance, manifest themselves in specific physical locations. Usually these sites are in relationship to the role of the transverse current in ordering the mind and emotions. For example, excessive worry normally resonates with the Abdomen current, physically affecting the upper digestive tract (especially the tissues of the stomach and duodenum), and may progress into an ulcerative condition. Energy vortices block and restrict the flow of the Qi, which eventually alters the directional flow of the Qi within the meridians and the transverse currents.

According to Chinese medical thinking, Qi normally invigorates the mind; yet emotions and thoughts are able to adversely influence the flow of Qi. Specifically, an imbalanced or excessive emotion will alter the flow of Qi; for example, anger causes the Qi to rise upwards; sadness and grief weakens the Qi; fear descends the Qi; worry stagnates the Qi; excessive jubilance scatters and slows the Qi; and fright disorders Qi.

The same phenomenon of altered Qi flow occurs with all the emotions. For example, mild annoyance, frustration, anger and rage form a sequential progression of emotional intensity, and they all elevate the Qi in a similar manner. Physically, when the Qi rises in anger, for example, the face flushes, the eyes glare, the voice pitch rises, the pulse quickens, the jaw locks and the muscles tense. In fact, even subtle thoughts produce changes to the Qi flow, but with lessened intensity.

When an energy vortex is contacted - either mentally, by experiencing a resonant feeling or thought, or physically by having awareness drawn to the site of a vortex - energy is released. The release of energy from a vortex produces a variety of mental impressions, emotional feelings, and physical sensations, and this temporarily abates its overall charge. In this way, there is often a state of dissipation and internal softening that follows a release. In time, however, the vortex again begins to accumulate energy because it absorbs the Qi that it blocks. Only through experiencing and healing its originating center can the vortex become divested of its energetic charge and its contents reintegrated into one's awareness so that Qi can flow freely through the tissues.

On a physical level these energy vortices occur primarily in the fascial tissues. They do, however, with time, penetrate into the surrounding tissues (muscles, organs, bones, blood vessels, nerves, etc.) when the fascia can no longer bear the restriction of energy that has built up. Eventually physical changes can occur within those tissues, thereby further impairing the Qi flow and predisposing an individual to a more serious medical condition.

Meridian Qi Revisited

Classically, meridian Qi is visualized as moving out from the chest to circulate along the meridian pathways. Meridian Qi appears to have a natural tendency to flow in a specific sequence and direction, probably being genetically encoded. Qi can, however, be made to move in any direction through intent or by disease. Voluntary conscious control of Qi and its movement can be mastered through utilizing the connection between the mind and the breath. This was demonstrated to me by Dr. Liu's mastery of the hot and cold needle effect, which I mentioned at the beginning of this chapter.

I envision the heart to be at the center of the whole meridian system. The physical medium of the meridian Qi movement is the fascia. The physical heart and fascia are both derived from mesodermal tissues. The meridian Qi's impetus for movement and the pace of the movement itself are, however, governed by the rhythmic motion of the heart and lungs. This rhythmic motion is a manifestation of an inherent somatic system. Nevertheless, the meridians are connected to the abdominal organs and embrace the brain and nerves. Below and above the heart, the endodermal abdominal organs and the ectodermal brain form the two other somatic systems. Thus the meridians interface with three somatic systems: the cranial, visceral and thoracic. This energetic affiliation between meridians and the threefold somatic system will be explained in the next chapter.

The meridian concept provides a valuable clinical tool for balancing and harmonizing the whole body. Often symptoms which are seemingly separate can be understood through the meridians as forming an integral pattern of illness. For example, once I had a pregnant woman, Kathy, referred to me by her midwife for a malpositioned fetus. She was 35 weeks pregnant, and the baby's head had not engaged itself downward. Kathy was worried because of the looming possibility that cesarean section would be used. According to the meridian theory we use a single point on the end of the fifth toe along the bladder meridian to treat this condition. Moxibustion is twice daily applied to the point, and usually within ten days there is a positive change. Clinical studies of thousands of women in China have shown an 85 percent success rate for this form of therapy. Kathy also complained about sinusitis, occipital headache, low back pain, mild incontinence and sciatica that had all emerged during the course of her pregnancy. According to traditional theory, all these symptoms were related to the bladder meridian's external route (western medicine would see these same symptoms as separate). In Kathy's case, within a number of days not only did her baby rotate and engage, but all her other symptoms cleared up as well.

Exercise 7
Circulating Meridian Qi

The purpose of this exercise is to sense and facilitate the flow of Qi within the meridians. In classical texts the meridians are described as follows: if you imagine a standing person with arms raised above the head, the Yang meridians move down the back and outside of the hands to the head to the feet while the Yin meridians move up the front and inside of the feet to the chest to the hands. Symbolically, the Yang meridians descend from the sky to the earth and the Yin ascends from the earth to the sky. Although the meridians are twelve in number, a precise knowledge of each meridian's route is unnecessary for this exercise. The meridian Qi flows under the skin just above the muscles in the superficial fascia, while deeper branches connect internally with the organs and tissues. The focus of this exercise will be on superficial meridian Qi circulation. Let us begin.

According to your comfort, assume one of the following positions:

1. Sit in an arm chair with your back relatively straight and comfortable, feet flat on the floor and the inside of your arms and palms on the chair's armrests.

2. Lie on your back on a relatively firm surface; you may choose to use a pillow under your head and knees.

Once you are in position, close your eyes and just sense how you are; make a mental note of any physical sensations, feelings or intrusive thoughts that may be apparent. Each step will be explained separately; then you can integrate them.

As you inhale, imagine Qi or energy moving from your finger tips down the backside of your hands, up the back of the forearms and upper arms, then over your shoulders into the sides of the head to your eyes. As you exhale, continue to move the energy from your eyes over the forehead, over the back of the head, down the neck, descending down the back and sides of your trunk, continuing down the back and sides of the thighs, legs and feet until the energy reaches your toes.

With your next inhalation, imagine the energy flowing from your toes around the underside and inside of your feet, up the insides of the lower legs to the inside thighs, continuing up through the groin into the front of the abdomen, then to the chest. With your exhalation, move the energy from out of the chest through the armpits, along the inside of the upper arms and forearm, then along the palms toward the fingertips.

You have completed a circuit of meridian Qi flow through two cycles of inhalation-exhalation. Repeat this sequence for about 10-15 minutes. Each time

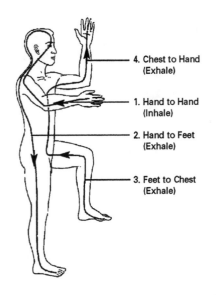

4. Chest to Hand
(Exhale)

1. Hand to Hand
(Inhale)

2. Hand to Feet
(Exhale)

3. Feet to Chest
(Exhale)

7-6 Circulating Meridian Qi

In summary, follow in order and repeat these steps: 1. inhale, while imagining Qi moving from the backside of your hand to the head; 2. exhale, continuing to move Qi from the head to the feet; 3. inhale, as you move Qi from the inside of the feet to the chest; and 4. exhale, while directing Qi from the chest to the hands.

allow your breathing and imagery to be more integrated so that a nice rhythm emerges. Remember to sense the Qi flow along the body's surface, just below the skin. If you have trouble visualizing the Meridian Qi flow occurring simultaneously on both sides of your body, then try focusing your awareness on one side for a while and then the other side before attempting to visualize both sides at once.

You may also have a tendency to breathe deeper when you do this exercise. This is normal. Allow yourself to soften the breath as the energy flows. Next time notice if you are using different parts of your lungs in the two phases of breathing, when the energy is moving toward the head (Yang phase) and when it is moving toward the chest (Yin phase).

After you have stopped the exercise, sense how you are. Notice if anything has changed in your sensations, feelings or thoughts. Slowly move about and pay attention to how you feel over the next few hours.

CHAPTER EIGHT

Somatic Organization and Rhythms

*"There is a primal force, but we cannot discover
any proof. I believe it acts, but I cannot see it. I can
sense it, but it has no form." - Zuang Zi*

Modern science has given us deep insights into the nature of things. We have been able to isolate, study and manipulate matter as never before. Our world has been transformed by a dazzling spectrum of new knowledge and technologies born from scientific discovery. For better or worse, electricity, automobiles, spaceships, vaccines, television, nuclear bombs, computers and other inventions have been bestowed upon humanity.

Nowadays, the rational and empirical approach, based on reductive thinking, is emphasized in nearly all institutions, not only in science but also in medicine, psychology, philosophy, economics and politics. In fact, the singular reliance on this approach has led to it becoming a virtual article of faith. In my opinion, the rational scientific approach has replaced religion in the late 20th century as humanity's repository of hope; it is commonly believed that by the pursuit of science a better and more just existence may be possible.

Yet science has nothing new to offer humanity as far as the big questions go, such as the essential meaning of existence and human life, or the source of creation and life on earth. Nor can it be said that the rational and analytical approach of science has given us any deeper understanding about human consciousness or the subtle dimension of human energy. For example, science has been unable to discern the relationship between brain and mind.

I believe that if you seek to know the intangible, you have to let go of the rational; you need to sense as well as to reason. I have observed that the intuitive, sensing and feeling parts of ourselves are much more capable of encountering and discerning the subtle realm of energy or the vastness of mind, or even the bliss of spirit. Reasoning is best left until after direct experience. Our ability to rationally think is not our most significant or smartest faculty. This is not a new idea. Zuang Zi, the Taoist philosopher, is also reflecting upon the intangible in the quote at the beginning of the chapter. He expressed those heart felt words about the inner life force more then twenty-five centuries ago. Today, as in the past, this real and vital experience of inner energy is accessible to all. We must, however, learn the art of "optimizing."

However, we need not reject the rational and analytical approach; rather we must nurture and trust and learn how to incorporate the constructive, intuitive, synchronistic and holistic ways of thinking and acting. In this way a true balance may be achieved in our perception and knowing that will allow the sensing and feeling parts of ourselves to flourish. Understanding and healing the whole person is a creative art. We cannot understand living forms by studying their material components alone; we must grasp their dynamic aspect, that which moves and gives life meaning.

Presently there is a renaissance along these lines occurring within the healing arts, from acupuncture to hands-on therapies to herbal medicine to psychology. The boundaries of our knowledge about the body, energy, and the mind are expanding rapidly. This expansion of knowledge is being driven mainly by direct experience, by practitioners who strive to explore beyond the limited concepts of the past. In time, rational explanations for many of these new insights may be possible, but for now many are beyond scientific proof. Until then, it is imperative to continue exploring the subtle realm. It has yielded many treasures. Let us take heart and move on.

In this chapter, the three fundamental somatic rhythms will be surveyed. These three rhythms reflect inherent energy systems. They are perhaps the most "gross" expressions of the energetic terrain, because they directly manifest within the physical body as observable patterns or rhythms. They are dominant coordinative forces which enable the physical body to function properly.

For some time now the existence of these somatic systems has been acknowledged, and physical proof of their existence has been anticipated. In particular, Rudolf Steiner (1861-1925), a renowned teacher and perhaps the last "renaissance man" of Europe, gave us many insights into the significance of the human body's threefold division.

Dr. Steiner had a deep breadth of knowledge and began a movement called Spiritual Science or Anthroposophy. His work led to the founding of many influential movements such as Waldorf education, anthroposophical medicine, biodynamic gardening, and so on. Steiner believed that the body is organized according to a threefold scheme. He observed that in both structure and function the nerve-sense pole of the upper body is opposed by the metabolic-movement pole of the abdomen and extremities; yet they are united by a central harmonizing element, the rhythmic-heart system found in the chest. Essentially, Steiner perceived a natural threefold organization; the upper and lower poles are opposite in nature while the middle is a harmonizing force.

Apparently, Steiner sought to both affirm and reinterpret the classical medical teachings of Hippocrates, Galen and Avicenna (980 - 1037 AD, known also as Hakim-ibn-e-Sina). The scope of classical medicine in the west was without doubt as holistic and profound as that of ancient China and India. Unfortunately, classical western medicine went into a steady decline with the advance of modern biomedicine not long after the time of Nicholas Culpeper (1616-1654), the famous English herbalist, astrologer and author of numerous books on classical medicine. Fortunately, Steiner breathed new life into these long forgotten teachings, in particular those of Galen. Galen taught that the life force (Pneuma) expresses itself in a threefold manner, namely, the "animal faculty" centered in the brain, the "vital faculty" in the heart and the "natural facult" within the abdominal organs.

I have reflected for many years upon Steiner's interpretation of Galen's ideas. I believe his insights into the threefold nature of the human body offer important clues about the organization of the energetic terrain. I found parallel ideas in many cultures; in particular the Chinese concept of heaven, earth and humanity reflects a similar image. The physical proof of the existence of somatic rhythms within each of these divisions (cranium, chest and abdomen) has also emerged, mainly through the astute research of a few osteopathic physicians. I believe these three systems and their rhythms do have an energetic foundation. They are part and parcel of our energetic terrain. I owe a great debt to the teachings of Steiner in pointing the way forward.

The Triune Energy Pattern

Earlier in this book, we have seen that within the psychoenergetic core the Vitality, Heart and Brow centers respectively anchor the physical, energetic and mental spheres. Furthermore, these same three centers within the core also help organize the transverse currents and embryonic vessels, which in turn facilitate the patterning of the embryo's three tissue types.

As I mentioned in Chapter 6, there occurs a process of polarization amongst the three primary tissues after the embryo's third week. This process is initiated by the transverse currents acting upon the embryonic vessels. Essentially, the endoderm tissues within the Anterior vessel migrate, accumulate and differentiate in the lower abdomen, while the ectoderm tissues within the Posterior vessel follow an opposite course, focusing themselves in the head. Thus, a polarity forms with the Yang-like ectodermal nerves in the head opposing the Yin-like endodermal gut in the abdomen. In between, the mesoderm tissues of the Middle vessel become diffused throughout the evolving embryo, although the physical heart, being mesoderm in origin, acts like a central hub for all the mesoderm.

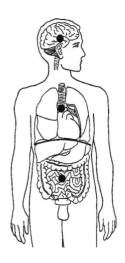

8-1 Three Somatic Systems

From above to below the three systems are as follows: the Cranial centered in the ectodermal nerve tissues in the head; the Thoracic where the heart acts like a central hub for all the body's mesoderm tissues; and the Visceral centered in the endodermal gut tissues of the abdomen. The three more-or-less equidistant dotes depict their approximate center of functioning and subtle motion.

Crucial to this whole process of polarization are the Vitality, Heart and Brow centers of the psychoenergetic core. They are the guiding forces by which this process occurs, as a result of the innate Yin-Yang polarization within the psychoenergetic core as a whole and the Yin-Yang polarity within each center. This polarized potentiate at the centers is referred to as subtle particles (bindus) in the Tibetan Tantra teachings. Essentially, the three centers set the subtle tone of each separate somatic system and its inherent rhythm. Thus, overall the combined influence of the psychoenergetic core acting through the embryonic vessels and transverse currents results in the manifestation of a somatic system and rhythm. The following basic relationships emerge-

Core		Vessel		Current		System
Brow	☞	Posterior	+	Head	=	Cranial
Heart	☞	Middle	+	Chest	=	Thoracic
Vitality	☞	Anterior	+	Pelvic	=	Visceral

Each of these three systems has its own unique manifestation of energy, inherent motion and physical form. They are closely related yet independent. They are like the visible spectrum of light, differing in color but connected in nature. Keeping to this analogy, the energies of the core, of the vessels and of the currents are outside this visible spectrum, being subtler in nature. Each system's inherent rhythm or motion is physically subtle but palpable by a trained practitioner. The physical form and rhythm of each system is centered around the seat of a primary embryonic tissue.

Together, the three somatic systems are a step-down in vibration or octave as compared to the three embryonic vessels and the transverse currents. Like the Qi that flows in the meridians, the somatic systems are closer to the physical body; they embrace and coordinate the tissues within their sphere. Of course, the three systems overlap both energetically and physically. In a healthy person, the somatic rhythms operate independently yet in harmony, like differing voices in a choir.

Using the Chinese model of essence, Qi and spirit, I believe that the lower abdominal or visceral pole is linked with the body's essence or biological force. The middle thoracic pole is associated with the Qi and the meridians they move through, while the upper nervous or cranial pole is reflective of the mind, a fundamental attribute of spirit according to Chinese philosophy. Appropriately, the Chinese refer to the archetypal image of heaven, man and earth to depict this relationship between spirit, Qi and essence within the threefold division of head, chest and abdomen, respectively.

Threefold Structure and Function

A number of interesting observations come to light when we view the three somatic systems from a physical perspective. Practically, the differences between the upper and lower poles manifest in their differing rates of rhythm. The inherent cranial motion is slightly more accelerated (8-12 cycles per minute) in comparison to the visceral motion (6-8 cycles per minute). The thoracic rhythms are of a different order altogether. On average for an adult, the heart beats about 72 beats while the lungs respire about 18 cycles during each minute; a four to one ratio. Also, the cranial and visceral motions are harder to detect, since they are subtler than the more apparent thoracic motions.

Structurally, the bones of the skull constitute a solid envelope surrounding the soft internal parts. Conversely the abdomen consists mainly of soft tissue that is freely exposed to its surroundings; its hard bony structure is relegated to the back and sides. In between the rib cage of the thorax is a flexible amalgamation of hard and soft tissue.

Functionally, the nervous system is the center for sensory absorption, integration and interpretation. We see, hear, smell and taste directly through the senses in the cranium. As well, we organize our ability to move and sense touch through the brain. On the other hand, the abdomen is where we receive the physical nourishment from food and liquids for our survival. We assimilate, metabolize and discharge wastes through the healthy functioning of the abdominal visceral organs.

The metabolic processes of the lower visceral sphere are concerned with building up the body. We are connected to the outside world physically through the abdominal organs. What we take in as food and drinks from the world around us are continually being absorbed and transformed within our abdominal organs. Our bodies are a reflection of what we consume. The nerve-sensory processes of the upper cranial sphere involve the consumption of nutrients and grosser energies such as calories and oxygen. We are also connected to the outside world through our senses and awareness. We absorb information into our heads, while in our abdomens we absorb material formations.

In both structure and function, the nerve-sense pole of the upper body and the metabolic pole of the abdomen are united by a harmonizing element, the neutral system found within the chest. The function of this intermediary system is to reconcile the opposing forces of the nerves (which consume energy and do not regenerate, a disintegrative tendency) with the digestive tract (which absorbs energy and is involved with tissue renewal, a regenerative tendency).

Psychologically, the upper nerve-sense system is the instrument of thought, through which the senses are ordered. The lower pole is that of movement, metabolism (which is subtle movement) and exchange. The entire metabolic system is the instrument of will, our ability to physically survive. In harmonizing the upper and lower, in forming the bond between thinking and willing, the thoracic system is the instrument of feeling.

The heart is the principal organ of the thoracic system. The heart should be considered not only a mechanical pump for blood, but also as a restraint, by virtue of its ability to put rhythm into the blood flow, which can be felt in the pulse. Embryologists have long known that blood circulates in the human embryo well before the heart beats or even appears. I believe that the meridian system, in which Qi flows, is energetically connected to the heart and lungs and through them to all the other organs and structures within the body. This is why feelings are so closely connected to the movement of Qi.

The above differentiation of this threefold somatic system needs to be seen in the context of a diverse physical body. The physical tissue types associated with one somatic system will be present in the other two systems. For example, the nerve-sense capability that predominates in the cranial pole will be present as a secondary influence, as nerves, in the thorax and abdomen. Thus all three systems and their rhythms may be felt anywhere in the body, if you can attune yourself to them, just as you would a radio frequency.

In my understanding, the limbs rely on all three systems for proper functional and structural balance. They depend on proper nerve force, nourishment and movement and ability to rhythmically and gracefully move respectively from the cranial, visceral and thoracic spheres.

In the following pages I would like to explore each individual somatic system, especially the new insights from osteopathy, a form of physical medicine which advocates structural balance. Osteopathy utilizes joint and soft tissue manipulation, postural reeducation and other physical therapies to treat a wide variety of disorders. The present day practice of osteopathy in America has veered more towards conventional medicine in its thinking. Only a determined minority of osteopaths are still advocating the use of manipulation and the body's ability to heal itself.

The Visceral Organs

The body's organs are considered the foundation of the body's metabolic processes from a biomedical perspective. For quite some time medicine has known every organ's main physiological features, secretions, anatomical shape and so on. Medicine has developed sensitive instruments to analyze, and theoretical models to understand, organ pathologies. Yet medicine is not so effective at treating functional disorders, such as, for instance, dysmenorrhea, chronic fatigue, arthritis, depression and asthma. In my experience, most functional disorders emanate from the mind and energetic terrain, leaving medicine poorly equipped to deal with these ailments. As a result, functional disorders often become chronic in nature. This situation is like a car that has everything in order structurally, but still it does not perform well. The car needs to be tuned and functionally integrated before it is road worthy.

In all systems, whether they be energetic, physical or mental in nature, imbalances arise from an alteration to their inherent function and/or structure. Both aspects -

function and structure - must be taken into consideration when treating or analyzing the causes of disease.

One overlooked phenomenon within the body is the inherent motion of the organs. Motion and rhythm are characteristic of all living things, including the bodily tissues. In the last twenty years the study of inherent organ motion has mainly been done by French osteopathic physicians, notably Dr. J. P. Barral, a developer of a unique form of visceral manipulation. Dr. Barral and associates crafted a model of organ dynamics based upon two features: their biomechanical movement and inherent motion. He called these, respectively, organ mobility and motility. In Barral's innovative work visceral manipulation is applied, using biomechanical principles, to correct organ dysfunctions. To confirm their theories, Barral and associates documented changes in the viscera before and after treatment through the use of x-ray fluoroscopy, ultrasound and infrared emissions.

Anatomically, organs are enveloped by fascia and separated by serous fluid which provides protection and lubrication. The organs have a sliding surface which allows for a certain amount of mobility to occur in response to the body's movements, especially the diaphragm's piston-like action. For example, Barral has estimated that the kidneys have an amplitude of 3 to 4 centimeters in response to one cycle of inhalation and exhalation of the breath. This range of motion of the kidneys is repeated with each respiratory cycle, over 20,000 times a day, to a total of about 600 meters of movement daily. Naturally, restrictions to mobility can cause serious functional problems to the kidneys or reflexively to other organs and adjunctive structures like the vertebral column or blood vessels. In fact, visceral restrictions can have consequences throughout the body, giving rise to numerous conditions, such as headaches, varicose veins and depression.

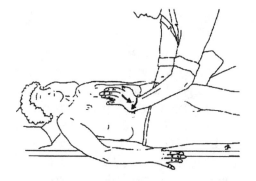

8-2 Kidney Technique

In the above illustration the visceral practitioner is performing an induction technique to balance the right kidney. The arrowed lines on the practitioners hand shows the right kidney's intrinsic movement or motility during the inspir phase.

Besides the biomechanical mobility described above, organs also have an intrinsic motion or motility which has important energetic implications. Apparently, all organs have a subtle rhythmic motion with two phases, passive and active, just as in breathing. Organ motility can be perceived with training. According to Barral's research, the motility of a specific organ mimics the migratory movements during an organ's embryonic development. Embryologically, the budding organs first appear during the fourth week. Their positions are not fixed in the rudimentary gut; rather they migrate around for a number of weeks. I believe, as others do, that within all the tissues there is not only inherent motion but also inherent memory at work.

The theory of visceral organ motility postulates that motion occurs around a point of equilibrium. An organ alternates between an accentuation of embryonic movement and a return to its neutral position. In general, organs tend to move towards or away from the midline-navel area, which seems to be the focal point of inherent motility. The movement towards the navel (expir) is the relatively passive phase while the movement away from the navel (inspir) is the more active phase. Normally, this phasic organ motion occurs synchronistically amongst all the organs. Motility has three chief components: amplitude or range, rhythm, and vitality. Motility directly reflects the functional capacity or energy of an organ.

Chinese Medicine and the Organs

According to Chinese medicine, the organs are invested with both essence and Qi. The function of the organs is to maintain and nourish the essence which manifests on a physical level as wholesome nutritive blood and reproductive tissues (ovum and sperm). Qi is the functional capacity of the organs to perform their role. I believe that visceral motility is a manifestation of organ Qi. However, in general, the Chinese concept of the organs is different from modern medicine's.

Nevertheless, both Chinese medicine and modern bio-medicine do agree that the organs have biological rhythms. These rhythms are marked by periodic, fluctuating levels of organ activity during different times of the day. Functional or circadian rhythms have been known to western science, especially with the investigation of syndromes related to rapid long-distance travel, wherein the body's biorhythms become disturbed. Circadian literally

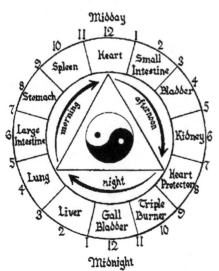

8-3 Chinese Biological Clock

This diagram shows the times of the day and their related organs according to Chinese medicine. During each period of time the corresponding organ and meridian are believed to function at their optimal level when healthy. The inner triangle represents the three-fold division of the day that begins with an organ of the chest - lung, heart and heart protector (i.e., pericardium) - which are the hub for all meridian Qi activity. In their own way western science is just beginning to research and apply the knowledge of circadian rhythms to the practice of medicine.

means "time periods in a day" and refers to biological processes that occur regularly within a twenty-four hour time period.

In Chinese medicine, the various biological rhythms of the organs are reflected through and harmonized by the meridian system. As mentioned in the previous chapter, the meridian system helps amplify the external terrestrial and cosmic influences. In this way, man's inner rhythms are linked to the external rhythms of nature.

I have found that this knowledge of organ rhythms can throw light on illnesses that follow predictable patterns. For example, insomnia in which a person wakes up consistently around 3 o'clock in the morning is usually due to an energetic blockage between the liver and lungs, while a collapse of physical and mental vitality after lunch, around 1 or 2 o'clock in the afternoon, is usually due to a small intestine problem. Furthermore, in my experience, a disturbance in an organ's motility or mobility is usually the cause of an organ's dysfunctional circadian rhythm.

Once I was treating a patient for a severe urinary problem. Bill had a frequent and urgent need to urinate, sometimes four or five times an hour, but little urine came out and often voiding was painful. Typically, his problem was aggravated during the late afternoon, a time of day that in Chinese medicine is linked with the bladder and kidney's biological rhythm. During one session, as I manipulated his kidneys, he suddenly broke out in a sweat and starting to cry uncontrollably, feeling a great outburst of fear. Bill sensed electrical-like charges, the Qi, being released deep within from his kidney towards his bladder and penis. His abdomen and lower back started to heat up and to relax as the Qi started to flow through the area. Needless to say, his condition rapidly improved after that, healing completely in time.

The Cranium

In the early 1930's, an American osteopathic doctor, W.G. Sutherland, after twenty years of investigation, announced his discovery that the cranial bones move, and that there exists an inherent perceptible rhythm within the cranium. He termed this previously unknown motion the cranial rhythmic impulse, or CRI. Conventional anatomical teachings at the time stated that the cranial bones were immovable, their sutures being more or less fused in adulthood. Sutherland's pioneering observations formed the basis of a new treatment approach for cranial dysfunctions.

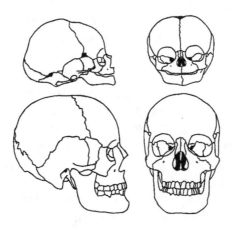

8-4 Newborn and Adult Cranial Bones
The cranial bones of a newborn are normally highly flexible and free to move so that the head can easily contour to the birth canal. Over time the skull bones thicken and grow toward each other to form sutures and joints. Ideally the cranial bones remain free to move, if only slightly, so as to accommodate the internal inherent motion and whatever external force that may be encountered. Thus the sutures in the adult skull are by nature designed to offset the subtle movement of bones just as faults along the earth's crust offset the subtle movement of its plates.

Sutherland believed that his therapy is applicable for a wide range of disorders both within or outside the cranium. Just as in the visceral system, cranial restrictions are thought to impact upon the adjunctive tissues and have far reaching consequences throughout the body.

The osteopathic concept of the cranium is based on a number of observations, primarily: a) that the brain and spinal cord, as a functional unit, have inherent motility; b) that the cerebrospinal fluid circulates and rhythmically fluctuates; c) that the cranial bones move; d) that there is a significant reciprocal motion in the sacrum which occurs in response to cranial movement; and finally, e) that the cranial motion is transmitted throughout the body via the fascia.

The CRI is composed of two phases, referred to as flexion and extension. The impetus for the motion occurs within the cranium. Considering the head as a whole, flexion involves a slight transverse widening of the head, while its anterior-posterior dimension shortens. Extension is opposite to this, involving a transverse narrowing and an anterior-posterior lengthening of the head. In response to the cranial motion, the sacral apex (the end adjoining the tailbone) moves anteriorly during flexion and posteriorly during extension. The whole body also responds to the CRI, producing a rhythmic pulse wave, palpable throughout the body.

In the 1970's, researchers at Michigan State University, headed by Drs. Upledger and Vredevoogd, established the scientific validity of cranial bone mobility. Their research results largely supported Dr. Sutherland's basic tenet, although they differed on the question of the source mechanism behind the CRI. Dr. Sutherland believed that the initial impetus for the CRI was the brain and spinal cord's inherent motility, which causes the cerebrospinal fluid to fluctuate and cranial bones and membranes to move. He postulated that the embryological coiling of the neural tube continued as a patterning force within the adult brain and spinal cord.

The Michigan State University team proposed an alternative, the pressurestat model. They proposed that the rhythmic fluctuations of cerebrospinal fluid are paramount and form the driving force behind both membranous and osseous motion. In the Michigan State model, cerebrospinal fluid production is automatic; the fluid's input-output production is dependent on neural receptors in the sutures between the skull bones, particularly the sagittal suture along the top of the head. Also, they emphasized the importance of the dural membranes. The pliable dural membranes conduct the cranial motion to the sacrum and, via the fascial system, throughout the body. In fact dural membrane is a type of fascial tissue. Dr. Upledger utilized this perspective to develop innovative techniques, under the name Craniosacral Therapy, which emphasizes the restoration of mobility of the dural membranes and fascial system.

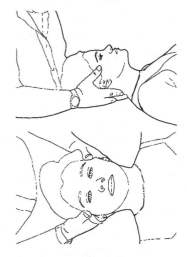

8-5 Craniosacral Technique

This illustration shows a craniosacral practitioner applying a vault hold with his hands, a technique that can be used for both assessing or treating cranial distortions.

The cerebrospinal fluid is considered by many osteopaths to be the highest and most pure substance within man, regarding it as essential to proper nervous system functioning. Indeed, Dr. Sutherland, in his lectures on cranial osteopathy, often referred to an invisible element, the "Breath of Life," as giving potency to the cerebrospinal fluid. This potency was envisioned by Sutherland as originating from a higher source, having been inspired by a passage in the bible: "And the Lord God formed man of the dust of the ground and breathed into his nostrils the breath of life and man became a living soul" (Genesis 2:7).

Embryologically, the cerebrospinal fluid first appears in the deep recesses of the developing brain, called the ventricular area, from which it will actively assist in regulating the ongoing production of cerebrospinal fluid. This fluid carries no waste products, only pure nutrients that irrigate the tissues of the brain and spinal cord. Research has shown that the cerebrospinal fluid migrates in small quantities down the optic and auditory nerve sheaths. These two sensory organs and structures are more or less of ectodermal origin. I believe cerebrospinal fluid acts both as a conductor and accumulator of energy for the nervous system.

Interestingly, Galen, the previously mentioned Greek physician and father of western classical medicine, believed that the inherent motion of the ventricles in the brain propelled the life force (Pneuma) residing within the brain throughout the body. The life force within the brain was considered a distinct emanation and was referred to as the "animal faculty." He believed that as the ventricles fluctuated in the brain the "animal faculty" life force is transmitted down the nerves into the body.

The Taoists also have similar ideas that strikingly resemble the above craniosacral concepts. The Taoists mention two esoteric structures, the jade pillow and the sacral gate, which transmit Qi. Physically, the jade pillow is imagined as being situated within the brain, anterior to the occipital bone at the back of the head. The sacral gate is thought to be located within the sacrum. They help to circulate Qi within the extraordinary vessels and connect the upper and lower Fields of Influence. Specifically, the sacral gate is said to draw in and elevate the Qi upwards, while the jade pillow, in the head, circulates the Qi within the brain.

From a developmental perspective, the sacrum and occiput are the last two bones to fuse (in early adolescence or early adulthood), thus perhaps revealing their pivotal role in circulating Qi and organizing physical development.

Still-Point Phenomenon and Energy Release

An important phenomenon, both in cranial and visceral therapy, is the manifestation of a "still-point" effect. This occurs when there is a temporary cessation of the inherent rhythm in either one of these systems. By inducing a still-point, the targeted organ deeply relaxes, readjusts, revitalizes and discharges excessive or blocked energy, if necessary. Usually, a still-point affects the whole body, producing a softening of the breath, relaxing of muscle tone, and harmonizing of various physiological processes. Sound, music and meditative states that perfectly resonate with the brain or a visceral organ have also been shown to induce a still-point. In a healthy person, blocked or excessive energy can discharge itself from the body whenever necessary. For example, such releases often occur during a spontaneous still-point or when one is falling asleep. The experience involves a sudden jerking sensation of the body, followed by deep relaxation.

Sometimes a release of energy during a still-point can have an emotional quality or hold mental impressions attached to the physical and energetic release. For example, Carmen had come to me for her severe sinusitis, which had been bothering her ever since she could remember. I found, among other things, her cranial bones to be very tight and restricted in a number of places, especially in the right temporal area. I used a combination of cranial manipulation and acupuncture to treat Carmen's problem, as well as her underlying constitution.

During the third session, as I held Carmen's head, she entered a very deep still-point. She started to gently cry and tell me about the images that had entered her awareness. Carmen saw herself as a little girl, perhaps four or five years of age. Her mother was saying how bad a girl she was and she saw her mother's hand hitting her on the head. Carmen again felt a deep pain arise and slowly release. She remembered that the hitting did not happen just once, but many times over. She had never recalled this before, but now she understood that her sinusitis had started back then, in reaction to the physical abuse by her mother. Carmen also recalled that her mother stopped hitting her after the sinusitis appeared. Perhaps, Carmen offered afterwards, her mother's own feelings of guilt about her sinus trouble was the reason for the physical abuse ending.

The Thorax

New light has recently been shed on the workings of the physical heart which alters the notion of the heart as a sophisticated pump. Scientific researchers in the emerging field of cardio-energetics now believe that the heart acts as a main coordinator and communicator of energy and subtle information. From their perspective, the heart is viewed as a highly complex sensory organ that constantly monitors the individual's wellbeing. Numerous studies show that the heart is able to communicate and at times synchronize with the brain and other parts of the body via its intrinsic nervous system, hormone (atrial naturetic factor), and other pathways. By exploring its electrical, magnetic, acoustical and thermal emissions a complex picture is emerging of a heart which subtly influences not only our bodies, but our thoughts and feelings as well. Given time, I believe this avenue of research will reveal more of the energetic connections between organs and perhaps even of their subtler sustaining energies such as the transverse currents.

Energetically, the heart is the cardinal organ of the thorax. The lungs are its lifelong companions. Together they act as a mediating force within this threefold energetic system. They reconcile the forces above and below, in the cranium and abdominal viscera. The movements of the heart and lungs are grosser and more noticeable than the subtler cranial or visceral motions. Perhaps subtler motions exist within the thorax, but surely they are overridden by these more apparent rhythms.

As in the cranial and visceral spheres, the organs of the thorax are enveloped by fascial tissue, such as pleura, pericardium, ligaments and linings which provide structure, protection and support. As I have already mentioned in the previous chapter, I believe the meridians of Qi are dependent on the fascial tissue as their medium. The meridians take advantage of the numerous fascial connections to infiltrate every region of the body. The meridians provide the essential interconnections between all the three somatic systems. They are, however, governed by the thoracic rhythms, heartbeat, and breath, which sustain the circulation of Qi. I do not know the exact origin of the meridians, but I suspect that they evolve in conjunction with the limbs, after the appearance of the heart, in the embryo.

According to my experience, the general principles and techniques of both craniosacral and visceral manipulation can be applied to the thorax because they both work with fascia. But, primary amongst techniques for influencing the thorax is acupuncture, which can regulate the Qi and blood flow.

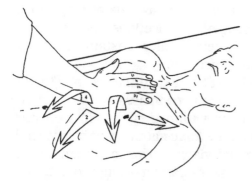

1. Lung, Superior Pleura
2. Inferior Pleura, Abdominal Organs
3. Heart
4. Gastroesophageal Junction

8-6 Thorax Technique

A practitioner performs local listening, a subtle method of diagnosis used in visceral manipulation. The arrows point to areas of possible restriction or tissue tension when the hand is drawn in their direction.

In Chinese Medicine, the thorax is considered to be like a central station or axis for the distribution and circulation of the Qi. Furthermore, Qi is said to move the blood, while refined aspects of blood help to vitalize Qi. Therefore, a reciprocal relationship exists between Qi and blood, as between the heart and lungs.

Although the thorax is neutral in polarity, if we compare the two organs, the heart is more Yang in nature while the lungs are more Yin. The heart is considered Yang because normally it manifests a faster and stronger rhythm compared to the lungs which have a softer and slower motion. Furthermore, the heart moves and paces the blood whereas the lungs absorb Qi from the air, in the form of oxygen and other subtle elements useful to the body.

I believe the rhythms of the heart and lungs are harmonized by the Heart center of the psychoenergetic core, acting through the chest current. Strictly speaking, the rhythms of the heart and lungs cannot be separated; they are interdependent motions. In fact, the body's pulses reflect the primal unity of heart and lungs, through their agents: blood and Qi. This is why Chinese medicine emphasizes the importance of pulse diagnosis in assessing disease. When a person is healthy and relatively in balance, the pulse will appear harmonious and full of vitality. Illness arises when the mind or body becomes disturbed. Thus a change in the flow of Qi and blood leads to a corresponding qualitative change in the pulse.

In my experience, the problems that manifest within the chest are usually due to disturbances outside the thorax, from the nervous system, above, or the metabolic system, below. Problems that originate within the thorax especially the heart are often more serious in nature, the result of a congenital defect or deep emotional trauma.

Without doubt, the mind is a potent force that can directly alter the flow of Qi and blood, and the rhythms of heart and lungs. Since the thoracic motions are more noticeable, it is relatively easy to consciously regulate our breathing by focusing our attention. We can also master skills to control our heartbeat and blood pressure, but this is a more challenging endeavor. Modern day biofeedback and visualization techniques or ancient yogic practices have been shown to alter the heartbeat and blood pressure. Understandably, the cranial and visceral motions are more difficult to influence with the mind, since they operate silently beyond our awareness.

The mind is dependent upon the nerve-sense pole above, for its ability to interact with matter, whereas the blood and essence are reliant upon the metabolic pole below to sustain matter. In between, the Qi which enlivens matter is subject to the influences of the neutral thorax. Breath and Qi are interdependent for the maintenance of life. When we are born we breathe in; when we die we breathe out. Breath is the visible form of Qi that silently sustains life. Without Qi there is no breath, and without breath Qi would collapse. They are interdependent.

A number of years ago, while I was in Chile, a patient came to me. Between my English and his Spanish, Jorge explained that his main concern was an utter and painful shyness. Jorge was in his mid 40's and he lived with his mother. He had never been in a relationship with a woman, something that he deeply wanted. Jorge felt himself to be awkward and withdrawn, being incapable of opening himself up. His physical health was excellent and his mind was sharp. He was an accountant by profession. In my assessment I found that his pericardium was energetically blocked. In Chinese medicine, the pericardium, or lining of the physical heart, is known as the heart protector (xin bao). The heart protector is imagined to function like a gate for the heart, allowing the inner self and feelings to flow outward and that of others to be received inward. Jorge's pericardium was blocked and I do not know for certain how or when this began. However, I did have a lingering suspicion that his relationship with his mother played a strong role in shaping the situation. In treatment I applied acupuncture, about once a month. In a little while his personality began to change; he started to reach out and share feelings with others. Jorge eventually started a relationship with a woman, his heart had started to heal, and he decided to live on his own.

Recognition of Systems

Our life force is present in our embryonic development, fetal growth, birth, childhood, adolescence, adulthood and old age. It accompanies us throughout our life cycle until death. Then and only then does the life force or energy dissolve, allowing the physical body to return to the elements. The three somatic systems are integral features of the energetic terrain. They are intimately linked to the health of both mind and physical body.

The three somatic systems and meridians lend themselves easily to assessment and treatment. They lie closer to the physical sphere. On the other hand, the psychoenergetic core, embryonic vessels, and transverse currents can be assessed by a skilled practitioner, but they are more difficult to influence in the short term.

I believe a working understanding of these somatic systems is an essential requirement for knowing how the mind and body operate. In my clinical experience, the recognition of the somatic systems has been an invaluable tool in working with illness. Indeed, I have sought to integrate my understanding of the energetic systems and the various healing modalities that I use to influence them into a coherent approach, one that I call Somatoenergetics. In this way, I believe that I have become more successful in working with my patients. I am also better able to impart to my patients and students the interdynamics of the mind, body, energy, and spirit. I feel that I have not reached nor hope to ever reach the end of my learning. This is the joy in the art of healing.

I do hope that this outline of the somatic systems will serve as a beginning for your own investigations.

Exercise 8
Sensing Subtle Rhythms

The primary purpose of this exercise is to experience the subtle biological rhythms that are being driven by the energy of the somatic systems. In this exercise try not to differentiate what you are sensing; just let your mind focus on the motions that manifest. Later on you can analyze what you have felt.

To perform this exercise you will need an inflated small round balloon. The 10" size is preferable. The balloon's function is to provide an inert but movable barrier, so that the hands and arms will be able to amplify the internal rhythms. The balloon does not have any internal motion, but you can sense your own rhythms that are conducted down your arms and hands through the balloon, through your kinesthetic awareness.

Throughout the body, subtle movements are constantly occurring. The cranial, visceral and thoracic rhythms are continually being emitted from the depths of our being. I find it wondrous that we can perceive and isolate each rhythm within the human body by touch alone.

Let us begin the exercise. First find a comfortable chair or stool. You may want to sit forward near the edge of the chair so that your back is free and you have more elbow room. Place your feet flat on the floor and allow your spine to be straight but relaxed. Your elbows and arms should be away from the sides of your trunk. The elbows are bent and the hands are out in front with the balloon (knotted end facing away from you) in between the palms of your hands.

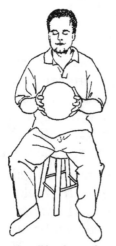

Try to hold the balloon so that the palms and fingers are in full contact with the surface of the balloon. Ease off any pressure that you may be exerting on the balloon. Minimum tension should be felt in your hands or arms.

Now concentrate your awareness on your hands and arms. Take a few

8-7 Sensing Rhythms through Ballon

184

deep breaths in and out; at the same time notice how your hands move in relation to the breathing. There will be a slight expansion and contraction felt on the balloon's surface, as if the whole balloon is moving. Slowly quiet your breathing while maintaining awareness of the perceived breathing motion on the balloon. Let this perceived breathing motion fade into the background, while your awareness remains alert and calm. Wait until you can sense another rhythmical motion pattern emerge. Most often you will start to sense a slower pattern coming into your awareness. Whatever emerges, try to stay with it. If you have difficulty sensing anything new, try gently and slowly to push your hands together against the balloon. Use minimal force. Then release and follow the balloon out. Try to pick up on any new motion. Repeat this last sequence if you need to. Once you have a new motion, stay with it for a couple of minutes.

As you are sensing, make a mental note of the newly found motion's rate. There may be a difference in duration between the expansion and contraction phases. Now, for a few moments, alternate focusing your awareness between your breathing pattern and this new rhythm. You can play around with your breathing by gently changing its rate, at the same time monitoring the motion in the balloon. But do not breathe too deeply or withhold your breath. Determine if the rhythm perceived by the hands is stable in spite of any changes in breathing. If the rhythm felt by the hands is dissimilar to and unaffected by the breathing, you have tapped into a subtler motion.

Normally, the cranial motion is between 8 - 12 cycles per minute while the visceral motion is a little slower. The breathing cycle is around 18 per minute and the heartbeat about four times as fast. Generally, most people will tap into the cranial rhythm first. The visceral motion is more challenging to sense in the hands, but it is possible. Occasionally, a person may tap into even subtler energies, such as the meridian Qi flow. They will have an even faster oscillating motion. Try to ignore the faster motions and concentrate on the grosser rates.

I have found this exercise helpful in teaching my students about energy and the somatic systems. You may wish to perform this sensing exercise from time to time in order to attune yourself to the inherent motions of the overlapping energetic and physical spheres.

CHAPTER NINE

Healing Concepts and Meditation

*"A man is born gentle and weak, at death he is
hard and stiff. Green plants are tender and filled
with sap, at death they are withered and dry.
Therefore the stiff and unbending are the disciples
of death. The gentle and weak are
the disciples of life." - Lao Zi*

So far, we have explored the structure and function of
the energetic terrain from a perspective of its relative
integrity and balance. However, as we all know, ill health
and an incomplete sense of well being and vitality often
afflict us. The energetic terrain, lying in between the mind
and body, plays a crucial role in our pursuit of healing
and wholeness. In this chapter, I would like to explore
how the energetic landscape becomes imbalanced and
how the various energetic systems can be restored to their
proper functioning. I will mention a number of the specific therapeutic techniques. These will be further described
in the Resource Guide to Some Recommended Healing
Arts, later in the text.

Energetic Blockages and Communication

In Chinese medicine, there is a saying: where there is
pain there is blocked communication; where there is open
communication there is no pain. The Chinese concept of

pain, as reflected in the Chinese ideogram, includes pain of both physical and mental origin. Significantly, acupuncture considers its primary purpose to be that of maintaining a free and flowing communication within the mind and the body. I am certain that Qi is the leading facilitator of mind-body communication.

In my opinion, not only is blocked communication the primary cause of disorder within the energetic terrain, but all healing techniques and therapies should be judged on their ability to enhance communication, whether within ourselves, with others, or in our relationship to the world. Inherently, blocked communication is blocked energy.

In general, blocked energy arises from either or both the mind or physical body. Whether the source was mental or physical trauma, habitual dietary indiscretions, an emotion such as fear, living outside of nature's rhythms, the day-to-day stresses in one's life, or something else, ultimately an energetic blockage is created. The blockage may be very subtle in nature, affecting only the psychoenergetic core, if, for example, a deeply held karmic pattern is involved. Blockages can also manifest on a grosser energetic level, for example, affecting the cranial system following a traumatic head accident. Unless resolved, blockages do in time become more problematic and are often sites where energy vortices evolve, as previously discussed.

Pain is the main indicator that an energy blockage exists. Pain can be very subtle in nature, such as a feeling of anxiety, worry or mild distress, or it can be very physical and extremely debilitating, such as the pain from a fractured bone or wound. Pain is the mind's and body's way of drawing awareness to an area in need of healing. Sometimes, awareness of pain becomes suppressed when survival is at stake or when the survival instinct becomes distorted by chronic unconscious emotional patterns such as fear and shame. These emotional patterns are usually potent and habitual in nature.

Ideally, no matter what form of practice or therapy is used to treat a blockage and restore balance, the patient's own active participation should be sought. A person can actively participate by focusing upon and integrating the mental, emotional or physical impressions that arise in a healing session. These impressions usually arise from the tissues where there are energy blockages or vortices occurring. By consciously becoming aware of the mental, emotional and physical impressions, followed by their acceptance and integration, the underlying blockage can be completely released. Generally, this does not happen all at once but rather over time while focusing on that particular blockage. In this way, the karmic seed or originating pattern of a blockage, once integrated into awareness, can be avoided in the future. Otherwise, only a temporary alleviation in the symptom pattern is obtained which, later on, results in the reappearance of the same or more intensified blockage, or the reemergence of that blockage in a transmuted form, with differing symptoms and/or location.

The principle of blocked energy and vortices has been demonstrated to me by innumerable patients over the years. One patient, Fred, clearly showed me the mind-body's ability to generate and then heal a profound energetic restriction. Sadly, later on within the same area of the body the blockage reemerged in a different form because the root cause had not been eliminated.

Fred came to me suffering from a deeply distressing inability to swallow. He had found no relief or satisfactory explanation for his problem from regular medicine. The doctors had tried drugs and surgical dilation of the esophagus with balloons to stretch it out; these approaches only gave him temporary relief, and the problem kept on getting worse. His esophagus was severely narrowed, and over a couple of years' time his food intake became reduced to semi-solids taken through a straw. Emotionally, Fred was blocked in his ability to communicate with and express love to others, including his wife and children. For many years he had been an alcoholic and I am sure he tried to drown his sorrows in his drinks. Looking at this situation from an energetic perspective, I believed his awareness was blocked at the Throat and Heart centers of the psychoenergetic core. Perhaps there was some originating trauma or karmic seed for all of this. I don't really know, but this man was suffering and slowly dying from his inability to nourish his body and soul.

I started to give Fred acupuncture and his whole outlook on life began to change; his swallowing improved and so did his ability to express himself. After a few months of regular treatments, he awoke one night and started to cough violently and up came a six centimeter long cigar-shaped tumor from his esophagus. The next day he came in and showed me his prize. Not only did he feel great but now his swallowing was more or less back to normal. I congratulated him and suggested we continue for a few more sessions. During those last few treatments I talked to him about what the underlying root issues of his esophagus problem might be. I suggested counseling and perhaps doing some art or music therapy to get in touch with and really heal that deeper level of himself.

As so often happens, however, Fred decided all was well enough, and he just wanted to carry on with his life. It's interesting that his medical doctor had refused to do a biopsy on the tumor or even to believe that it had come out of his throat. About five years later Fred suddenly developed cancer of the throat, which began in the esophagus and rapidly spread throughout the tissues in that region. He died within a couple of months. I had kept in touch with him, mainly through his wife, over the intervening years, and the reemergence of the energetic blockage was not a surprise to me, although its intensity was. I saw Fred a few more times before he died, and I was able to give him acupuncture, which helped with his pain and eased his transition into the spirit world.

The Art of Healing

Healing is not an exact science, but rather is an art in which intuition, compassion and knowledge are all essential. In my experience, knowing where to start treating the energetic terrain is as crucial as the type of therapy applied. Usually, we have many sites of blocked energy within the body, which may or may not display symptoms. Ideally, the best results will be obtained when we recognize and address the primary blockage first. Generally, primary blockages are those that have the greatest intensity or amount of blocked energy. These restrictive blockages originate from an underlying physical or psychic disturbance that is directly related to the patient's problem, although they are often obscured by other symptoms. This is where a therapist's intuition is important.

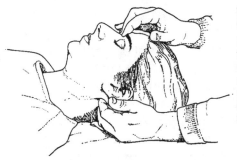

9-1 Releasing the Cranium Technique

Hands strategically placed at the sites of blocked energy will eventually allow for its release. In this technique the practitioner is gently holding affected acupressure points on the patient's head.

As energy is liberated through the release of a blockage, mind-body communication is enhanced and the patient's self-healing ability is increased. In a sense, all healing must be self-healing, since a therapist cannot force a person's energy to remain unblocked. The person's own work is fundamental to true healing.

In certain circumstances, such as in the advanced stages of cancer or when cancer arises in a devitalized and physically weak individual, directly releasing blocked energy may be inappropriate, because to do so could aggravate the condition. The main problem in these situations is that, in releasing the primary blockage, the person's mind-body awareness focuses on the cancerous tissues and energy is released from the tissues. If the person is already severely devitalized, there may not be enough energy and willpower to create healing. The energy will then be reabsorbed by the cancerous cells, further aggravating the condition. In this situation there are two main options: palliative measures, to help stabilize the mind and body so as to extend both the quality and length of life; or indirect methods (such as diet, cleansing, spiritual healing and so on) to revitalize the whole body, in this way trying to turn the disease process around.

Naturally, acute conditions such as a torn muscle, infection, fever, or an illness due to an emotional crisis take precedence over disease patterns that are longstanding. In these cases healing should be directed to those sites as needed, leaving the chronic symptoms and their underlying energy restrictions for later.

In my own practice, I use various hands-on diagnostic and therapeutic techniques for working with energy, usually with good success. However, I do refer my clients to other practitioners when my expertise seems inappropriate for the patient's level or type of blockage; for example, when healing a deeply held emotional pattern is the primary challenge, or when surgery is the obvious choice. I also believe the role of a healer is to help assist and encourage a patient's innate ability to know the meaning of one's illness and the best means to heal.

Over the years I have found that my work has become more gentle and less intrusive. Facilitating another person's energy flow does not require great effort, but it does require great sensitivity. You can gently turn on a light switch with your finger, or you can take a hammer and whack it to turn on the light, but you may damage what you have just whacked in the process. The same is true in our own energy system. This is what Taoists mean by softness overcoming hardness. This attitude is most helpful not only in my practice but in my life as well. Lao Zi's reference to the gentle and yielding as the disciples of life, at the beginning of this chapter, is true for both our body and our mind.

Below, I give some general thoughts and suggestions for balancing the various systems within the energetic terrain. I encourage those interested in working with energy, for yourself or in helping others, to train with an experienced teacher in whichever discipline you choose.

The Visceral, Cranial and Thoracic Fields

Within the energetic terrain, the three extensions of the embryonic vessels and transverse currents- the visceral, cranial, and thoracic systems - are closest to the somatic level. These three systems are, therefore, easier to manipulate, and the resulting changes will impact directly upon the energetic and physical spheres. In order to learn to feel the distinctive energies of these systems, training under an experienced practitioner is necessary. An important concept for perceiving energy (both its form and rhythm) at this level is called melding, a technique by which the therapist attunes to the patient's body.

Melding is like the musical concept of entrainment, in which two slightly different sounds start to resonate or vibrate as one. The clarity of perception that can be achieved by refining one's sense of touch and kinesthetic awareness through melding is truly astonishing. The key in the beginning is learning to differentiate which energy pattern you are sensing. At first all the rhythms may be felt together or only fleetingly, and thus discernment is difficult. But eventually one learns to differentiate the motions into their separate rhythms. This is like listening to a whole orchestra playing: with experience it is possible to differentiate each instrument's sound and contribution to the whole. Luckily, each system has its ideal listening posts for sensing the inherent rhythms in a person, and this makes the task of discernment easier.

The abdominal viscera are closest to the biological maintenance level of the human body, and as such they respond best to physical stimulus. Physical manipulation and massage, special diets, Ayurvedic purification therapy, physical exercise, deep breathing, botanical medicines, essential oils and potentized mineral preparations are extremely useful for healing the visceral organs. Chanting and the use of appropriate sounds are extremely valuable tools for unblocking and rebalancing these organs. As well, deep relaxation and a healthy routine are essential in treating any visceral imbalance. Following a regular routine and relaxation re-establish the normal circadian rhythm of the body and, in particular, the visceral organs. Of course, routine should be modified according to the individual's constitution and with consideration to one's surrounding environment.

The cranial system, being directly related to the nervous system, is intimately linked with the welfare of the mind. To influence the nervous system, massage is of particular value. Nerves and skin are of the same ectodermal origins and thereby maintain a strong resonance with each other throughout life. Besides, the skin is one big sense organ itself. Also, the use of music and color therapy is very effective for altering the nervous system. The eyes and ears, which receive sound and light, are a direct extension of the nervous system. These two sense organs serve as useful diagnostic and therapeutic openings into the brain. Sound, at the right frequency, has been shown to entrain and temporarily suspend the cranial rhythm to produce a still-point. Furthermore, gentle craniosacral or spinal manipulations are able to restore functional and structural balance to the nervous system and its environment. Prayer and meditation on geometric designs or mandalas can also be of benefit.

An important principle of Yoga is that energy follows the mind. What you think and concentrate upon directs the flow of your energy. The more freedom your thoughts have, the less blocked the energetic system becomes. As mentioned before, wherever energy is blocked, there probably exists an underlying feeling or thought in need of releasing. Techniques that work on the kinesthetic awareness are an effective form of refining and integrating the mind with the nervous system. This includes the use of psychophysical disciplines, such as the Feldenkrais Method, certain forms of Hatha Yoga, and dance movements. For best results, nervous system retraining should not be goal oriented. Forced movement, stretching and trying to achieve an ideal posture usually increases musculoskeletal resistance and reinforces existing nervous system patterns.

The thoracic system involving the heart and lungs is closely linked to the maintenance of overall energetic balance between the abdominal organs below and nervous system above. Often, structural and functional disorders that manifest within the chest are in response to what is occurring above or below. Therefore, looking at the whole situation is crucial when it comes to chronic heart and lung problems. As mentioned previously, the organs of the thorax also have a direct influence over the meridian system near the body's surface. In my opinion, the most powerful and efficacious method to restore balance in the thorax is through balancing the Qi within the meridian system. Direct hands-on manipulation and breathing exercises have also proved valuable aids in treating thoracic problems.

Furthermore, this heart-lung complex resonates intimately with and helps regulate the emotions and dream state. Any spiritual or psychological practices that promote love and forgiveness will, I believe, help heal the emotions and integrate dreaming within ourselves. Love and forgiveness are key steps which allow us to face and resolve the deeper, more complex patterns that await us in our journey to wholeness.

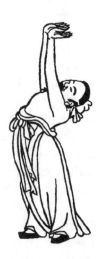

Techniques such as biofeedback and visualization can also have a profound healing effect upon the tissues and rhythms of the chest. As well, physical exercise is beneficial for the health of the heart and lungs, especially those exercises having rhythmic forms of motion, such as Tai Ji Quan, Qi Gong, dance therapy, and swimming.

9-2 Ancient Tao Yin Stretching Figure

In ancient China, Taoists promoted therapeutic exercise for health, longevity and spiritual attainment. The above drawing is based upon an illustration in the *Mind's Mirror For Preserving Life* (Bao Sheng Xing Jian), a Taoist text written in 1506 AD.

The Meridian System

In my experience, the meridians are particularly useful for releasing and harmonizing thoughts and feelings and, of course, treating physical concerns. In particular, the meridians can help to energetically balance and physically integrate the rhythms of the viscera, thorax and cranium. However, the initial effect of balancing the meridians is to harmonize the heart-lung relationship within the thorax. In this way the meridian system has a great influence over the whole body, having a harmonizing effect similar to the psychoenergetic Heart center.

Comparatively, within the energetic terrain, the meridians that convey Qi are like branches of a tree, while the psychoenergetic core is its roots and both the embryonic vessels and transverse currents form the truck.

The meridians spread themselves over the surface of the body and connect with the internal structures (organs, bones, muscles, blood vessels and so on). Through an understanding of their routes and internal connections, a great variety of symptoms previously seen as separate phenomena can be seen as an interlocked pattern. For example, a pattern of right shoulder pain, angry disposition, testicular pain, indigestion and a sore big toe may indicate a blocked liver meridian or disturbed liver organ. In my practice, this knowledge has helped me to clarify the underlying source of many chronic conditions.

I believe the most efficient and dynamic way to balance the meridian system is through acupuncture, which involves the needling of various points along the energetic pathways. In certain circumstances, other techniques can also be extremely effective to release the meridian Qi, such as the application of infrared laser light, finger pressure, heat or even gemstones on the points. The conscious (or unconscious) intent of the practitioner is important in guiding the outcome of this form of therapy. For example, those practitioners who believe acupuncture is only a physical therapy will produce different reactions than those who utilize acupuncture for psychological problems. This quality of intent can be mastered with proper insight and training.

The Embryonic Vessels and Transverse Currents

Generally, as we move closer to the psychoenergetic core, the energetic structures become less accessible to direct physical intervention. In the energetic terrain, the embryonic vessels and transverse currents lie midway between the psychoenergetic core which borders and merges into the realm of the mind, and the three somatic systems of the viscera, cranium and thorax which extend into the physical body. The embryonic vessels and transverse currents can best be accessed, revitalized or released through techniques that work with the mental and energetic spheres, for example, by the use of visualization, prayer, and breathing techniques.

Specifically, for the embryonic vessels, directly imaging them through such methods as the Taoist microcosmic orbit meditation is very potent. I have described this mediation at the end of Chapter 5. The Taoists use similar special breathing sequences and visualization to release and invigorate the energy within the transverse currents. More physical approaches can, however, also affect the vessels and currents. Acupuncture, in my experience, is a good example of this, although skill and profound knowledge is needed to consciously work with these systems using this method.

The transverse currents are closely allied to the body's fascial segmentation and defensive protection. Often, excessive tension or somatic guarding are generated within those related tissues. Therefore, the use of hands-on therapies that work on the fascial and muscular tissues, such as Craniosacral Therapy, Jin Shin Do, Polarity Therapy, and deep-tissue massage may be useful in releasing blocked energy at this level. I have found that emotions and mental memories usually manifest with released energy when working with the transverse currents.

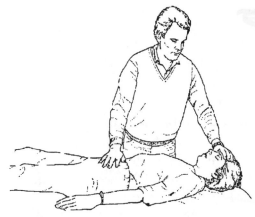

9-3 Integrating Heaven and Earth Technique

With one hand on the forehead and the other on the lower abdomen the practitioner attempts to restore balance between the upper and lower energies. This is a type of polarity technique used in Chinese massage to, metaphorically speaking, restore harmony between heaven and earth.

The aura is the farthest extension of the transverse currents. I usually use the aura for diagnostic purposes. For more information on how I use the aura, please see the exercise at the end of Chapter 6. I do not believe it lends itself to treatment since it is the outcome, not the source, of imbalance. However, directing energy through it to the tissues and energy within the body may yield results.

Compared to the transverse currents, the embryonic vessels, being connected with the human temperaments, resonate closer to the somatic level. Therefore those therapies, such as Ayurveda, that focus on regulating an individual's unique temperament are ideal. In my experience, the embryonic vessels are closely associated with physiological brain functioning. Simply put, the embryonic vessels set the physical parameters of the body (i.e. temperaments) that impact upon the brain's ability to function; thus the mind is influenced. Abnormal behavioral patterns, such as drug addictions, eating disorders, alcoholism, neurosis, schizophrenia and so on, often have at their root a disorder in the embryonic vessels. Treatment that incorporates dietary and lifestyle changes, along with medical intervention to harmonize a person's constitution, is the most effective approach to behavioral disorders. Acupuncture, specifically, is known to stabilize the mind during the withdrawal process in addictions.

The Psychoenergetic Core

The most profound level of the energetic terrain is, of course, the psychoenergetic core. The core embraces the psyche and pure spirit that touches upon the deepest karmic level of our existence. We can become gradually aware of the contents of the psychoenergetic core through spiritual and psychological practices, such as meditation. At times, awakening the psychoenergetic core and its seven centers may happen synchronistically with outer events or forces. I believe that these awakenings are always deeply personal and not necessarily the result of the outer events. Rather, they are in response to them and are what we call "triggers."

To my way of thinking, even practices such as laying on of hands, psychic channeling, so-called chakra balancing, spiritual healing, the use of gemstones, and so on do not directly affect the psychoenergetic core. Rather, they activate and release the primary energy fields within the energetic terrain, such as the meridians, cranium, or viscera; perhaps they even affect the transverse currents and embryonic vessels. Releasing these outer energies may in certain situations, however, impact upon the psychoenergetic core. Normally, though, the core is reached through inner intention and through the expansion of awareness. This process allows awareness to incorporate the contents of the personal and transpersonal infraconscious that are stored within the core. This is akin to the individuation process Carl Jung spoke about.

It is possible, however, to enter the psychoenergetic core effortlessly and without conscious intention if a person is inwardly ready. Spontaneous awakenings of the whole core are rare. Usually only certain aspects of the psychoenergetic core are brought into one's awareness at a given time. Yet each of us always remains in touch with this level of our being, although we do not know it, through our nightly descent into sleep.

Sometimes awareness can be projected into a super-sensory world in which contact is made with the psychoenergetic core through the use of certain psychotropic drugs such as LSD, peyote and yage. This can be extremely dangerous, though, if the person is not prepared for or guided into that realm, since the mind can distort or severely repress its experience when normal awareness is resumed. I am convinced that through psychotropic drugs many people unintentionally expose themselves to psychological trauma because they are not ready for the impressions and images projected out from the infraconscious realm.

In my practice, I use intuitive methods to try to comprehend the state of my patient's psychoenergetic core. By this, I mean the nature of their mind and spirit as well as the karmic restraints that they may be burdened with. This often helps me to understand the cause of their illness. I do not pretend to treat, heal or alter a person's core; only they can do this. But sometimes I am fortunate to be there when it unfolds. However, I can suggest ways to "self- heal."

To make contact and understand our own individual psychoenergetic core, I believe meditation offers the safest and easiest route. Meditation is a powerful tool, not only for spiritual development, but for mental, emotional and physical healing. Unfortunately, most meditators are not fully aware of the effects of their chosen practice. If it is true meditation, it provides clear awareness.

The Art of Meditation

In meditation there are three fundamental modes of concentration, each with its own effect. These modes are: active concentration on a fixed point of reference, whether internal or external; visualization or guided imagery wherein the mind focuses on a moving image sequence; and the maintenance of a non-focused awareness. Each mode of concentration is linked to the mind through the psychoenergetic core. The primary function of meditation, no matter in which mode, is to instill a presence and attitude of peace, a modality of being, which is meant to be carried over into every moment of one's life. Ultimately, the attitude of the meditator forms the essence of meditation and transcends the mechanics of concentration and other techniques. Still, differences in the three primary modes of concentration have an effect upon the experience of meditation itself.

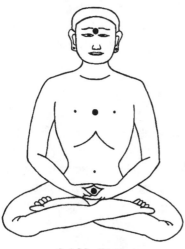

9-4 Meditation

Active concentration involves one-pointed attention on an internal or external object. For example, this technique is used for meditating internally on a sound, mantra, chakra or part of the body, or externally on a candle flame, mandala, a particular deity or guru. Internal light, sound and images arising within the mind's eye in the higher states of meditation are actively concentrated upon with single-minded focus. The object is to enter into a state of samadhi (at-oneness) and divine rapture by transcending mind and body. This form of meditation is performed under the auspices of the Brow center, in the head. Generally, the experiences that derive from Brow centered meditation are transcendental in nature, linked to the aspect of heaven, which frees consciousness to identify with the state beyond form and physical reality.

The passive, non-focused forms of meditation are utilized in mindfulness techniques, such as the Buddhist practices of Vipassana and Zen, as well as in the Taoist method of quiet sitting. Trance inducing music, such as shamanic drumming, is another way to enter the non-focused meditative state. In these techniques, the mind is simply watched without attachment or active concentration. This is similar to light dreaming, wherein a distance is created between the mind and its thoughts. Adjunctive techniques, such as the awareness of breath and/or returning the mind to an awareness of the body, help create the right internal ambience. In this regard, the lower abdomen is a natural place for the mind to focus upon, just as in sleep when the mind naturally withdraws into the lower centers of the psychoenergetic core. Through passive mindfulness there naturally arise ego-dissolving experiences of oneness. This state is also akin to the state of "divine surrender" that a devotee aspires to in Yoga. This devotional surrender involves a blissful and graceful letting go of one's effort and desires. Generally, this type of meditation is linked to the Vitality center, associated

203

with the earth aspect, through which oneness is felt as a syntonic connection to reality.

Visualization forms of meditation are common to Tantric and Taoist practices, as well as to a number of Christian forms, such as the Catholic meditation on the sacred heart of Jesus. Imagery also plays an important role in praying. For example, in the visualization of the boddhisattva Avalokiteshvara (who is called Guanyin in Chinese and Chenresi in Tibetan), an internal image of that deity is created, followed by projecting the deity's radiant light from the Heart center to all of creation and back. At the same time a prayer or mantra is normally recited. These forms of visualization are helpful in engendering feelings of universal love and compassion for the purpose of healing the meditator's psyche or healing others.

Visualizations, through their profound effect on the mind, are also helpful for healing the physical body. For example, when one feels love or imagines a loved one, that love is often physically felt to be in the heart, and all the other muscles relax in resonance to the heart's muscles. Love radiates out to the whole body, freeing deeply held armoring. Visualization incorporates both active and passive awareness, thus offering a balance between one-pointed attention and non-focused mindfulness. Ideally, visualizations are best performed through the neutral field of the Heart center. Metaphorically, the Heart center is representative of humanity, residing between the heaven and earth poles within the psychoenergetic core. Through this center, the self becomes submerged and loving identification with other people is made possible.

Effects of Meditation

The three modes of meditation differ in their resonance within the psychoenergetic core. Connection to the primal unity with life is made through non-focused awareness, centered in the Vitality center. Pure identification with humanity is achieved through visualization, connected to the Heart center. The transcendental realms of total detachment from mind and body are attained by deep one-pointed concentration, under the auspices of the Brow center. These three meditative approaches are symbolically represented by the images of heaven, humanity, and earth that are respectively linked to the Vitality, Heart and Brow centers. All three approaches are complementary in spiritual practice, since focusing on one meditative form alone can sometimes generate energetic blockages.

Generally, meditation is inappropriate for those people suffering from psychosis. In this condition, the mind cannot regulate, distinguish or fully integrate the impressions and images that arise from the infraconscious realms. In psychosis, the individual's normal barrier between the conscious and infraconscious realm has somehow been made permeable, and the dream-like world of archetypal images floods one's wakeful awareness. Thus, for the psychotic there is no protection from being pulled wide awake over the threshold into the image-filled world of the infraconscious. All of us experience this state in our nightly descent into sleep, but for most of us this barrier between the fanciful world of illusion and reality is solid. Carl Jung once said: "The mind does not oscillate between right and wrong, but between sanity and insanity." Meditation's main effect is to open up and integrate, in a controlled way, this deep level of the personal and transpersonal infraconscious which is beyond the physical senses and logical aspects of mind. Therefore, incorrect "meditation" would only weaken the barrier and further alienate the sufferer of psychosis from everyday life. Real meditation integrates, empowers and exalts consciousness.

The ultimate danger of wrong meditation is that it can bring out latent psychosis. In many societies preparatory work is given to those aspirants of meditation to prevent the chance of going mad. Moral regulation, selfless service, exercises to strengthen the individual's will and mental discrimination all play an important part in laying the groundwork for serious meditative practice.

Whenever meditation is done excessively, incorrectly, without clear understanding or with harmful intentions, certain signs appear. Each form of concentration has its own unique risks or side effects. Active concentration, which engages the Brow center, can result in a sense of detachment and a disassociation from one's own feelings or those of others, as well as upper-body symptoms such as headaches, hormonal imbalances, neck stiffness and a general lowering of the body's temperature. Passive concentration, which resonates with the Vitality center, can give rise to an inflation of one's ego, increased sexual desire, increased physical energy which may lead to irritability, and lower-body symptoms such as muscular and joint stiffness and pains, kidney and reproductive organ problems, and overheating of the body. Visualizations, which function best through the Heart center, can aggravate already existing emotional imbalances and attachments to others, as well as mid-body symptoms such as arrhythmia of the heart, chest pains, tremors and difficult breathing.

Ultimately, where the mind gravitates in our body will eventually manifest through our personality, whether consciously or not, whether in healthy balance or not. Even in modern speech the body's division into three regions is natural and implicit, such as when we say that a person "has guts" or "is kind hearted" or that they "live in their head."

In a general way, most societies have emphasized one of the above styles of meditation. For example, the Chinese and Japanese tend to utilize more non-focused techniques that involve the Vitality center; the Indians have emphasized more focused techniques that connect with the Brow center, while the Tibetans and Europeans orient their visualization practices through the Heart center.

Currently there is a trend in the western world towards synthesizing various traditional meditation techniques. Modern teachers, like Mantak Chia, Osho and Oscar Ichazo, each in their own way have attempted to integrate aspects of differing meditation traditions. Without judging these efforts, I believe that integrating the three forms of concentration offers a balanced approach for the science of meditation. Without doubt, meditation is a very positive tool to both awaken and heal the spirit. For each person, meditation should be tailored to suit his or her needs, without losing sight of maintaining the mind-body's balance.

Exercise 9
Cleansing with Healing Energy

I believe human beings have the capacity to draw upon cosmic and terrestrial energies to heal the self. Food, water and air are not the only elements that sustain life. They may be the basic necessities to maintain life, but they are insufficient to completely nourish our complex nature. Your mind is not cut off from your body. When you visualize something, not only does your brain respond to your imagery, but your whole body reacts. When we remember past experiences, it is not unusual for us to recall sensations and feelings, as well as thoughts. In this exercise you will be invoking and cultivating healing energy that is always accessible. By familiarizing yourself with this form of healing energy you will establish a new pattern and memory to draw upon. Various subtle energy systems will be engaged to accomplish this exercise, in particular the transverse currents. If you are ill or out of balance, practicing this visualization can be extremely useful. If needed, you may want to practice this exercise several times a day.

Begin by assuming a comfortable position, either lying down or seated. This exercise will take about 20 minutes. The spine should be relaxed and the arms and legs uncrossed. Close your eyes and tune into your body, allow your sensations to be present without trying to push them away; simply accept them. Next focus on your emotions, allow your feelings to be present and just acknowledge them. Do the same with your thoughts; just simply notice and accept whatever thoughts may still be present. Observe that you can separate sensations, feelings and thoughts within your awareness. Now, slowly begin to pay attention to your breath. At the end of each inhalation and exhalation, try to hold your breath for about two seconds; let this be a short comfortable pause. Continue doing this form of breathing for the next two minutes, then let your breathing return to normal.

Start to imagine a large orb of light above your head; award it a radiant, peaceful and healing nature. Gradually let it concentrate and spiral, like a funnel, down into the top of your head. When the light enters your head, let the light expand and bathe all of the inside of your head and right out to the skin's surface and sense organs. Again, perceive the qualities of the light: radiant, peaceful and healing. Slowly let the light descend into the next level, the neck. Again let this summoned light bathe and cleanse this whole region right out to the skin. After you have finished in the neck, descend through, one at a time, the chest, abdomen, and pelvis. Each time follow the same procedure as in the head: diffuse the light throughout that region.

After completing the pelvis, allow the light slowly to move down both of your legs. As the light descends, imagine the light radiating and flooding towards your feet. For a moment concentrate the light in the soles of your feet; then let it return upwards, ascending towards the pelvis. Keep moving the light right through the pelvis, through the abdomen into the chest. From there start sending it down the arms as you just did in the legs, slowly and unhurriedly until it reaches the hands. Once there, let it reverse and go upwards back towards the chest. From here, allow it to gradually diffuse throughout your whole body. Give thanks to this healing energy.

Slowly open your eyes. Notice any changes that may have occurred in your mind and body over the next few hours.

Journey's End

"I have suffered a sea change and nothing will ever be the same again." - The Tempest, Shakespeare

I have spent most of my life exploring energy for both healing and spiritual purposes. Yet I know there is still so much more to learn. This book was written knowing that there can be no final statement made about energy; until we know ourselves completely, energy will always verge on the mysterious. This book represents a beginning, a guide to the major energy patterns within us. I have only described the significant landmarks; there is still so much more to tell, know and experience.

The writing of this book has been a personal journey and a challenge. Originally I started this project in southern Chile, in the land of araucaria trees and majestic lakes, a most beautiful and isolated region. The book was completed here in Canada, a magnificent and spacious land, which lies closer to the pulse of our western civilization. During the last few years there have been many personal experiences and changes which have profoundly affected my life. Looking back, I see a great transition occurring, for I am no longer who I was and I have yet to become myself fully. Still, there is a certainty in knowing that I can continually reclaim parts of myself with each change that I undergo. I understand Lao Zi when he says that change is the only constant feature of life. Within myself, my feelings, thoughts and sensations are continually discovering change as I journey through life. For this I am grateful.

I also share in Jung's deep sentiment when he says "Life is - or has - both meaning and meaninglessness. I cherish the anxious hope that meaning will predominate and win the battle." Indeed, human life constantly mirrors a fundamental dualism; there appears within our experience not only meaning and meaninglessness but also beauty and cruelty, hope and despair, joy and sadness, pleasure and pain, love and hate, attraction and rejection, them and us, and so on. Each one of us experiences a separate version of duality playing itself out.

Today, we are facing a global crisis arising out of the human condition that calls into question our collective ability to live on this earth. It appears our arrogance and ignorance have allowed us to almost destroy that which we once thought to be so sacred and beautiful. I believe humanity must now choose a radically different mode of behavior and awareness, or else our survival on this planet is precariously in danger. We must search beyond duality.

During a recent trip to the Amazon I marveled at how nature embraces duality while simultaneously exuding a mysterious unity. On the one hand, the individual survival of plant, animal and human beings are weighed against a cooperative and inter-supporting relationship amongst all the elements and life forms of the forest. Order and chaos, life and death, meaning and meaninglessness coexist side by side in nature. Yet, behind or perhaps coming through all things in nature there is a presence, one that I have felt. This presence - whatever you want to call it - comforts and nurtures me, allows me to accept all that was, is and will be, allows me to feel at home. I sense it is great; all energy seems to unite with it. Somehow I know it is the source of all things.

Deep in my bones I know that my life is connected to all things. Once in Chile, on a warm evening in the fall, I was lying on the ground and I started to notice a deep, fathomless, but indescribably soft, breathing. It was slow and had a steady rhythm. I followed the sound until I was certain that this breathing was arising from out of a nearby volcano. I listened and submerged myself further into the sound, until my whole being resonated with each breath. I could feel the earth breathing from her core through the volcano into myself. Never have I been so touched by Gaia, our living planet and home. I am burdened by the fact that I can so easily forget these things. I feel heartened knowing that the unity of life is always within my reach.

I sincerely hope that this book will contribute to a growing acknowledgment of the wholeness of human life and nature. I hope there will be many journeys of discovery for you in the realm of energy. May you delight in the knowing and experience of your inner life force.

Taoism, Alchemy and Chinese Medicine

*"Knowing others is wisdom; knowing the self is
enlightenment."* - Lao Zi

Taoism is a coherent naturalistic philosophy that has
been an integral part of Chinese thought and civilization
for the last 2,500 years. Chinese alchemy is an extension
of Taoism, arising five centuries after Taoism's founding.
Alchemy advanced new methods for achieving spiritual
development and physical longevity, soon replacing many
of Taoism's earlier practices. Chinese medicine encom-
passes a broad scope of medical practices, all of which
subscribe to a rational view of health and disease. Over
time, Chinese medicine incorporated many of the theoretical and practical teachings of Taoism.

Together, Chinese medicine, alchemy and Taoism offer
a profound understanding of the human energetic structure. Their teachings come from a long-surviving and stable society with a rich history and literary tradition. Often,
governments gave official sanction and support to the
development and promotion of these teachings. Today,
each discipline is very much alive, not only in Asia but
throughout the world. The following concepts are presented with the aim of highlighting each discipline's unique
contribution to our understanding of the energetic terrain
and humanity's spiritual nature.

The Tao, Yin and Yang

Taoism believes that human beings can attain spiritual contentment and inner peace by living in accord with

the Tao. Practically, this means following and being in harmony with nature, for all of nature is viewed as a grand reflection of the Tao.

The word Tao denotes the primordial source of creation, which, although whole, has both a passive and an active aspect. The passive aspect of Tao is imagined as an unmanifest creative potential which gives rise to its counterpart, a manifest generative force. The passive and active aspects have been referred to as the Void and Great Ultimate. The active aspect generates all creation, continually binding it together, vitalizing it and allowing for continual change to occur, although the passive aspect of Tao remains unchanging. The Tao also instills each phenomenon with a unique characteristic which generates endless diversity within creation. Nature is the sum total of creation that human beings experience. The Tao is experienced both in the presence and workings of nature and the Void that lies beyond nature.

To a Taoist, achieving a life lived in harmony with nature involved following the intrinsic course of things, not by directing them. This is called non-doing. Lao Zi, who lived around 6 th century B.C., writes in the *Classic of the Tao and Its Way* (Dao De Jing)-

"In the pursuit of learning every day something is acquired.

In the pursuit of the Tao every day something is dropped.

Less and less is done until non-doing is achieved.

When nothing is done, nothing is left undone.

The world is ruled by letting things take their own course.

It cannot be ruled by interfering." - (Chapter 48)

In Taoist philosophy all of life exists in a state of duality and paradox. Duality means opposition and separation, as evident in day and night, cold and heat, anger and joy, life and death, male and female. Paradox means that these states are identifiable as separate only in their relationship to something else, since no phenomenon exists in absolute isolation. Taoism uses the words Yin and Yang to denote this idea of primal duality and paradox.

Originally the words Yin and Yang referred, respectively, to the dark and light side of a mountain. Later these terms were used by the ancient Chinese to express the concept of inherent duality within all things. Furthermore, there exists a dynamic tension between the forces of Yin and Yang that initiates a constant movement or process of change, causing Yin and Yang to continually unite, separate, regenerate and transform themselves. Yet their ultimate source remains in the Tao.

The earliest attributes given to Yin and Yang in the ancient oracle inscriptions are the receptive earth below and the creative heaven above. Later on, the analogies of water and fire were used to describe the intrinsic characteristics of Yin and Yang, respectively. This linkage also summarizes their qualities and differences. Below are the attributes associated with both of these forces:

Water	*Fire*
Yin	Yang
coldness	heat
moistness	dryness
dimness	brightness
stillness	activity
yielding	forceful
inhibition	excitation
slowness	rapidity
heaviness	lightness
downward & inward movement	upward & outward movement

The images of the Tao, Yin and Yang are vital components of the Taoist vision. They are simple yet profound aids that can be used to perceive and explain the natural ordering and laws of creation. The Taoist believes that an authentic human being is one who lives life in accord with nature, whose source is the Tao; to do otherwise means suffering and disharmony.

Early Taoism

The early followers of Taoism advocated the following three means in order to return to the Tao: the cultivation of inner wisdom by passive reflection; the gathering of awareness through mindfulness in one's actions; and by a deep observation of nature. In regard to the cultivation of inner wisdom, many Taoists prefer the practice of Quiet Sitting, through which communion with the inner source of the Tao is sought. They believe that in a non-active state, consciousness naturally returns to its root, the Tao. Thus no techniques are used in Quiet Sitting, for to do so would disturb consciousness. Only a mindful presence and a passive awareness is necessary, which differentiates Quiet Sitting from what happens in deep sleep. Being free of dream activity, awareness is absent, yet the mind has returned in tranquility to the apparent Void. This practice has striking resemblance to contemporary Zen and Chan meditative practices. On the other hand, awareness is believed to be naturally gathered through actions, whether mental or physical, that are performed with full alertness and in harmony with nature.

The Taoists also revered nature and observed her workings with great interest, for they felt that the mysterious laws of nature were the manifest workings of the Tao. They bestowed upon nature a nurturing feminine quality that reflects a feeling of intimacy achieved through deep insight.

Taoism and Alchemy

During the Han Dynasty (206 B.C.- 220 AD.) Taoism incorporated new ideas, many of them, no doubt, inspired by the arrival of Indian Buddhism and the new developments within the Chinese sciences. While adhering to the general principles of living in accord with the Tao, the Taoists of this period advocated the search for immortality and longevity. Their aim was to extend life to the absolute limit in order to create more time for practicing self-cultivation. This shift led to the development of alchemy, which may be defined as the manipulation of phenomena and time, to reach this objective.

Alchemy gave new impetus to the Taoists' investigation of nature and humanity. This research directly led to insights about the significance, structure and movement of energy within human beings. Active methods of life extension and self cultivation were developed which incorporated and exploited these new insights. As a result, during this era breathing techniques, chanting and the use of sound, physical exercises, meditations, mental imagery or visualizations, sexual practices and so on were all developed from Taoist alchemy. Often these new methods involved the harnessing of a disciple's intention and technical skill.

Generally, Taoist alchemy is divided into outer or inner practices, depending on the focus. Outer refers to the use of external agents to promote longevity while inner refers to the manipulation of internal substances and energies to enhance self cultivation. Most practitioners use both approaches, believing that they complement each other.

In outer alchemy, natural substances from the mineral, plant and animal kingdoms which enhance longevity are refined, transmuted and ingested. Historically, outer alchemy has been rightly referred to as a proto-chemical science, because it greatly aided the development of the natural sciences in China. For example, gunpowder was originally developed by the Taoists as a healing and life-enhancing agent before it was used in more sinister ways.

The Chinese interest in and search for an elixir of immortality was probably initiated by reports from India of a psychotropic plant called soma. This marvelous drug was first mentioned in the Indian scripture the Rig Veda, around the first millennium B.C. Soma was being promoted as a mystical substance that created visions, putting one in touch with the departed Immortals, or perhaps even creating them. One verse gives this description: When we have drunk Soma, we become immortal; going to the light, we found the gods.

On the other hand, inner alchemy concerns itself with what already exists: the human being. The purpose is to discover how to enhance, enliven and awaken all the subtle forces that operate within the mind and body. Like its counterpart, inner alchemy also promotes longevity as one of its goals. Yet, inner alchemy's primary purpose is for the aspirant to achieve an expansion of awareness so that the Tao can be perceived in full. Their focus was not on achieving mere physical immortality but on attaining spiritual immortality through a union with the Void, the passive aspect of the Tao.

The majority of practices in inner alchemy are centered around two closely related concepts, the three Fields of Influence and the three Treasures. The Fields of Influence refer to specific sites within the human energetic terrain, while the three Treasures refer to the principal subtle forces within embodied human life.

The Three Treasures

Taoists identify three principal substances - essence, Qi and spirit - which form the basis for the conception, growth and maintenance of human life. To honor their importance, these substances are referred to as Treasures. The alchemists believed that by enhancing and preserving these Treasures the health and well being of mind and body would be maintained.

The Chinese concept of spirit embraces the notion of an integrative force within consciousness which oversees the mental faculties of cognition, intuition, memory, discrimination, and so forth. The spirit is said to fully enter the body with the first breath, animate the body throughout life and depart from it with the last breath. The Chinese also perceive the existence of a soul that is part and parcel of the spirit. The soul is considered to be of multiple identity, having both material and ethereal parts that are related to the energies of the earth and heaven, respectively.

Qi is a more difficult term to define, a problem that most translators resolve by leaving the word untranslated rather then risking inaccuracy. Qi denotes the basic life force within human beings. It is visualized as a rarified immaterial substance that is on the verge of achieving form. Qi is differentiated into various types, depending upon its specific function, form or location. Take, for example, defensive Qi that circulates along the surface of the body, cosmic Qi that is absorbed by the lungs from the air, or liver Qi that refers to the specific functioning of that organ. Qi circulates throughout the body, communicating information and activating organic functioning through a system of meridians.

However, Qi is not limited to human beings. All things, according to their unique nature, are animated by an expression of Qi. On a cosmic level Qi can be seen as the materialized form of the creative tension that arises from the polarization of Yin and Yang.

Essence is representative of the biological matrix that determines human growth and development and ordains the unique physical characteristics inherent in each person's makeup. Essence, as compared to Qi, can be imagined as a rarified material substance on the verge of becoming formless. Essence is considered the matrix that forms the foundation of all tissues within the body. On a very material level, essence is most concentrated within the human reproductive tissues, especially the sperm and ovum.

The Three Fields of Influence

The Fields of Influence are sites within the body where the three internal Treasures can be gathered and transformed. The location of the Fields are associated with the middle of the head, chest and lower abdomen. The Fields are not considered physical structures; rather, they are energetic potentials which overlap the physical form. Around these sites a natural concentration of energy or Qi occurs which, when harnessed, facilitates the transmutation of the other Treasures.

In Chinese philosophy, the three Fields of Influence are related to the cosmological division of heaven, earth and humanity. The image of heaven refers to the powers of the stars, sun, moon, planets, air and sky. The earth is linked to the forces of the creatures, plants, oceans and lands of our planet. Man refers to the domain of human beings and their intrinsic energies. Within a person, heaven is used to denote the head and neck; humanity denotes the chest, and earth represents the abdominal region. As well, each Field of Influence is linked to a specific substance. These associations can be summarized as follows:

	Upper	*Middle*	*Lower*
Location	head	chest	abdomen
Aspect	heaven	humanity	earth
Substance	spirit	Qi	essence

First, in inner alchemy, the three Treasures are gathered then concentrated within the body. This is followed by the transmutation of the Treasures within the three Fields of Influence. This process proceeds in an orderly manner from the transmutation of essence into Qi, then Qi into spirit and finally spirit into Void, the non-manifest form of Tao. Perhaps, this concept of consciously directing matter so that it returns to the formless is difficult to grasp. But to the Taoists it is a real goal.

Specifically, the essence which naturally accumulates in the lower Field, located in the abdomen, is first transmuted into Qi. Then Qi is drawn upwards into the middle Field, within the chest, where it is gathered and transmuted into spirit. Next the spirit is made to ascend upwards to the upper Field, within the head, where it is concentrated, transmuted and, in time, dissolved into the Void. The process of upward transmission of the essence, Qi and spirit occurs along a mystical central vessel.

In ancient times, mental and physical techniques such as the practice of Tao Yin breathing and movement exercises were used to transform and transmute the substances. Tao Yin was a form of psycho-physical exercise which utilizes mental imagery, respiration and movement to create energetic change. The modern day disciplines of Tai Ji Quan and Qi Gong have their origin in this older practice.

Taoist Sexuality

Taoist alchemy's preoccupation with the preservation of the internal Treasures led to the emergence of a number of unique sexual ideas and methods. The Taoist belief that reproductive secretions are the manifest form of essence directly inspired techniques for men to forestall, diminish and if possible eliminate the loss of sperm during and after intercourse. For women, the loss of essence does not occur during intercourse, but rather mainly through pregnancy, childbirth and nursing, and only slightly during menstruation. Thus, special techniques were formulated for the female adept.

Ideally, for both sexes the potent force of orgasm is to be directed inward instead of being an outward release which dissipates physical and emotional tension. The significant lack of cultural shame associated with sexuality in ancient China no doubt facilitated their exploration of how to utilize this force. The Taoist teachings on cultivating sexual energy bear striking resemblance to similar practices in the Hindu and Buddhist Tantric traditions.

Chinese Medicine

Taoism and Chinese medicine share a long common history, especially during the formative period in their evolution. While Taoism is focused on the meaning of life, and how to achieve spiritual contentment, Chinese medicine concerns itself primarily with the maintenance of mental and physical well being. Traditional Chinese medicine views human beings as individually whole and not separate from nature. An understanding of holism permeates all the theories and modalities within this great healing art.

The pre-eminent text of Chinese medicine is the *Yellow Emperor's Inner Classic* (Huang Di Nei Jing). This classic was written during the Han Dynasty, a time of renaissance when both the medical sciences and alchemical arts flourished in China. The *Yellow Emperor's Inner Classic* expounds a medical theory based upon ideas drawn not only from Taoism, but also from Confucianism and shamanism as they existed in China at that time. This book laid out for the first time an integrative and logical approach to medicine, an approach based upon the following important theories: the Tao; Yin and Yang dualism;

the manifestation of five phases; and the concept of Qi and its circulation. From among the Taoist concepts, Chinese medicine adopted the understanding of the Tao and the Yin-Yang theory, as well as incorporating, from alchemical research, a number of ideas on the circulation of Qi.

The most important non-Taoist theory that influenced Chinese medicine was the theory of the five phases or elements. The five phase theory was first articulated by Zou Yin (350 - 270 BC.), a Confucian reformer who utilized the phases to describe the energetic links or resonances within creation, including human beings.

Fundamentally, the five phases are archetypes of nature and her forces, which the ancients intuitively felt. The five phases are denoted by the symbols wood, fire, earth, metal and water. The main energetic attributes are: wood is characterized by the process of germination and spreading out; fire has the emblem of heat and growth, with a flaring upward motion; earth represents nourishment and transformation, with an urge towards containment; metal is characterized by a maturing process and a concentrating influence; and water represents coolness, decay and storage, with a downward flowing motion.

The five phases are used in Chinese medicine to differentiate bodily structures and tissues, as well as to describe relationships between these and physiological or psychic processes. Thus organs, substances, emotions, bodily secretions, sensory organs, and external climatic influences can all be grouped according to their affiliation with a specific phase. For example, the wood phase is linked to the springtime, wind, the color green, the liver, anger, eyes, the shouting voice, and so on. This theory gives a powerful tool for understanding the origin and progression of disease.

Chinese medicine manipulated the concepts of the Tao, Yin and Yang, and the five phases to describe the functional relationships amongst the substances, organs and tissues of the body, as well as the mind or spirit. The study of disease origin and progression, diagnosis, prognosis, and therapy are all based on an integrative functional approach.

Therapeutically, Chinese medicine possesses a diverse yet complementary group of practices. Paramount among them is the practice of internal medicine, which deals mainly with preventing and curing illness through the use of plant, mineral and animal drugs. Next, there is the use of acupuncture, involving the piercing of the skin at specific sites with fine needles, and moxibustion, a technique of mildly heating the skin through the use of an ignited herb. Both acupuncture and moxibustion rely on a coherent understanding of the circulation of Qi throughout the body. Adjunctive techniques such as massage, manipulation, diet and remedial exercise are also a part of Chinese medicine's therapeutic tools. Nowadays some of these ancient practices have found a place within modern biomedicine, for example in the use of acupuncture analgesia in surgery.

Meridians and Vessels

Chinese medicine has a unique vision of energy, one that is based upon the idea that energy or Qi circulates along subtle pathways throughout the body. At the foundation of this energetic system are twelve meridians and eight extraordinary vessels.

The twelve meridians are the most accessible and superficial routes of Qi flow. The meridians provide a system of communication, defense, and connection between the body and mind and the surrounding environment. In addition they connect the surface of the body to the internal organs, which are said to store unique expressions of essence, Qi and spirit. Along the meridians are tiny openings or acupuncture points wherein Qi accumulates. At these points, therapeutic massage, moxibustion or acupuncture needling can alter the quality and redirect the flow of Qi.

The whole meridian system, according to the *Yellow Emperor's Inner Classic,* begins from the chest area and extends throughout the body in a systematic fashion. Normally, a complete cycle of the Qi circulation along the meridians and associated organs occurs over a twenty-four hour time period. The meridians are also divided into Yin and Yang divisions, depending upon their associated organ and direction of flow. If one were to visualize a person with hands extended above the head, the Yin meridians flow from the ground upwards through the chest to the hands, while the Yang meridians flow from the hands downward via the head to the feet. All the meridians orient themselves in a vertical direction, head to feet.

The extraordinary vessels are identified as being deeper and subtler than the regular meridians, having their origins in the human embryo close to the time of conception. These vessels are said to facilitate embryological development and organize the body's physical and energetic structure, including the twelve meridians themselves. Furthermore, extraordinary vessels are seen as reservoirs of the body's Yin and Yang potentials, as well as Qi and blood, which the meridians may draw upon in times of need.

In total there are eight extraordinary vessels described in Chinese medicine. These can be divided, according to their function, into three groups: the belt, the primary, and the secondary vessels. For more information on the eight vessels, see Chapter 5.

The Vessels as Psychic Conduits

To Taoist practitioners, the vessels are also seen as psychic conduits which regulate and communicate with the three Fields of Influence. An intimate knowledge of the vessels is considered to be extremely important for spiritual progress, longevity and well being. The meditative insights of the Taoist adepts and sages most likely inspired, if not developed, many of the theories relating to the Qi and its circulation. Undoubtedly their deep contemplative practices facilitated the Taoists' ability to perceive the subtle patterns within themselves and nature.

While Chinese medicine teaches that there are eight vessels, Taoists mention one other vessel, a mystical central vessel (zhong mai). This vessel is believed to directly connect and open into the three Fields of Influence. The mystical central vessel is closely associated with spiritual awakening and the transmuting of the substances, as previously discussed.

The Present

Unfortunately, Taoism has lost most of its importance in mainland China, mainly due to the rise of materialism and the influence of modern sciences. Sadly, while in China I saw and heard many stories about the suppression of Taoist beliefs and the destruction of sacred sites. Nowadays Taoism is only practiced by a small portion of the populace. But as of late, Taoist concepts have recaptured the attention of many people, both in the East and the West.

On the other hand Chinese medicine has fared better; it has entered into a period of renewal within China, and has been widely adopted and adapted by foreign cultures. Acupuncture has especially been successful in attracting attention from people in the field of biomedicine and the western public in general. The ever widening scope of available literature within this field is a testament to its new found success.

Appendix II
Yoga, Tantra and Ayurveda

"Lead me from darkness into light; lead me from untruth into truth; lead me from mortality into immortality." - Vedic prayer

India is both blessed and cursed by its vast array of religions, castes, cultures, languages and geographies. India has never been the land of one homogenous race. Rather, India absorbed each new set of conquerors and wandering tribes with their differing ideas. Each group, whether it was the Aryans, Muslims or British, all found themselves trying at first to convert the conquered, but with time, coexistence became the norm. These foreigners became more Indian with each generation and yet remain, even today, societies within a society. Hinduism, the largest religion in India, shares in this rich tradition of diversity. The variations in the beliefs, practices, deities of worship and philosophies makes Hinduism difficult to grasp.

The Indian Hindu tradition has given humanity three profound and fundamental bodies of knowledge: Yoga, which deals mainly with the spirit; Ayurveda, which focuses on the physical body; and Tantra, which is chiefly concerned with the mind. The philosophies of these three disciplines are basically in accord with each other; only their emphasis and practices differ. In Yoga, the body and mind are sought to be harmonized with the spirit. Ayurveda aims to balance the body and mind so that they are in agreement with the natural laws of the universe. Tantra seeks unity through expanding awareness and purifying the mind, while balancing the demands of the body and spirit. Yoga, Tantra and Ayurveda all ultimately direct the individual to go beyond limitations and achieve complete freedom and liberation from the "cycle" of births. They also share similar views on the nature and significance of the energetic terrain. What follows is an outline of the major themes of each tradition.

Yoga

Yoga is an ancient practice which has developed and evolved over thousands of years. The word Yoga means union, referring to its intent, which is union with the divine. The history of Yoga, like Tantra and Ayurveda, reaches deep into the age of the *Vedas* more then 3,000 years ago. The *Vedas* are a collection of hymns, written by rishis or seers of truth, that reflect the slow evolution of ancient Indian thought, from the worship of nature deities, with ritual sacrifice, to the use of soma, and eventually to a recognition of one absolute reality that is all-pervading and infinite.

Central to the theory of Yoga are the laws of karma and rebirth. Karma denotes action; the law of karma basically proclaims that every action or thought has a consequence, even if it is not immediately apparent. The present is a result of past actions and thoughts, and the future is dependent on one's present actions and thoughts, which generate new karma. Rebirth, or reincarnation in the Hindu context, is the belief that the individual soul or spirit, due to karma, will at some point after the death and dissolution of the present body be obliged to enter a new form. It is believed that all karma ultimately arises from thoughts and the illusory state of separation engendered by the mind. Thus the goal of Yoga is to still the fluctuations of the mind and body, and thereby enter a state free of thoughts, feelings and sensations, called samadhi.

As outlined in the *Bhagavad Gita*, the great spiritual gospel of the sixth century B.C., there are many forms of Yoga in Hinduism, each stressing a different practice to achieve union. Principal among these are the traditional Yogas of action, devotion, and knowledge. Later on there emerged another discipline, known as the Royal Yoga, which articulated an integrated doctrine based on older concepts and practices. This Royal Yoga was first formally codified in the third century B.C. by the rishi Patanjali, who fused the divergent yogic concepts with the essence of the Samkhya philosophy.

The Samkhya tradition teaches that our reality arises from the union of a transcendental awareness and an innate nature. This idea is parallel to the Chinese notion of the passive and active aspects of the Tao. Furthermore, according to the Samkhya tradition, nature expresses itself in three primal forces (gunas): inertia, activity and equilibrium. The three forces are proactive in generating five great elements: ether, air, fire, water and earth. Together the five elements form the material basis of all phenomena.

Patanjali's Royal Yoga contains eight steps that an aspirant must pass through and perfect on the journey towards divine union. The first two steps are practices encompassing ethical and moral restraints. The third is that of harnessing and stabilizing the body through physical postures. This step forms the basis for the practice of Hatha Yoga that is so very popular in the west. The fourth step is concerned with controlling the breath, which is seen as the physical reflection of the mind and energetic realm. The fifth deals with the withdrawal of the senses, so that the mind becomes still. The sixth concerns the development of concentration, or one-pointedness of mind. The seventh is meditation, the art of being able to merge the mind with the object one focused upon. The eighth and last is samadhi, the supraconscious state in which the influence of mind and body are withdrawn from the field of relativity and its forces to a field of pure awareness. In samadhi, the pure spirit delights in itself, thus entering into a divine rapture or union.

The ultimate result of the yogic process is a strong sentiment of detachment instilled into the adept's consciousness. The world is seen as a place to which the individual is bound by karma, a place to withdraw from in order to return to the spirit. Thus renunciation and asceticism have always been strong features of Yoga and Hindu culture in general. Tantra on the other hand does not seek withdrawal from life, but to transform consciousness and to heal the dichotomy between spirit and matter. For the disciple of Tantra, the goal is to achieve a synthesis through working with one's mind.

Tantra

Although Tantra is an ancient practice with roots in the Vedic age, it was never expressed as a concise discipline until after the second century A.D. The philosophy of Tantra hinges around the principle of non-duality between spirit and matter. Tantra tries to erase from awareness the tendency towards dualistic thinking, in which judgements exist about what is holy and what is profane. In order to achieve this, Tantra teaches that the universe is composed of two aspects as represented by Shakti, the feminine, and Shiva, the masculine. The feminine is considered the primal force within all of creation, while the masculine aspect represents the pure state of awareness or being. Both the feminine and the masculine principles are taught as being part and parcel of each human being. Tantra believes that the way to unite these two aspects is through retraining the mind's perception and interpretation of reality.

In Tantra the body is exalted, as is all matter, and special tools are used to retrain, expand and harmonize the mind. Most significant of these methods are: the use of prayer or mantra; visualizations or guided imagery; ritual worship of deities that personify forces within consciousness; meditation on sacred drawings or geometric designs, respectively called mandalas and yantras; the use of body postures and gestures; and the transmutation of sexual forces through rituals.

Five Sheaths

According to Tantra, in the human being there are five sheaths of differing vibrational density. The five sheaths are, from most dense to subtlest, as follows: the gross or physical sheath; the subtle life force or Prana sheath; the cognitive and discriminatory sheaths which engender the mind and individuality; lastly, the causal sheath of pure consciousness, which essentially is the repository of all one's karmas. Yet, beyond the realm of the five sheaths is a mystical dimension that embraces the undifferentiated, pure and immortal spirit. Often this last realm is referred to as the transcendental sphere (of the pure spirit).

In the human body all these differentiations, from the material body to the subtlest level of spirit, occupy the same "space", just as the different frequencies of sound (from audible to inaudible) co-exist within the same field.

Understanding reality and the nature of mind is fundamental to Tantric pursuit. In practice, Tantra emphasizes the feminine principle in worship and mental training. The feminine force is believed to manifest in the form of vital energy throughout all of nature. Within human beings, this force is called Prana. The tantric adept endeavors to harness and transmute Prana in order to reconstruct and purify consciousness. First, the inner Prana is stabilized, then potentized and ultimately redirected inward and merged with the subtlest levels of the mind. In the last stages of the inner tantric journey, one-pointed awareness and concentrated Prana are utilized to contact and activate the latent feminine force within, referred to as the kundalini. Once this latent energy awakens, it is said to move through various psychic channels within the subtlest sphere of energy.

Subtle Sphere

Tantra developed a model of the energetic sphere that was later adopted by Hatha Yoga. According to the Tantric model there are numerous channels called "nadis" in which Prana flows. The concept of the nadis and Prana are remarkably similar to the Chinese description of the vessels, meridians and Qi. The most important channel is the sushumna, a central channel along which are situated a number of energetic centers called chakras. The sushumna and chakras are considered extremely subtle, so subtle that they are normally imperceptible to the senses. The latent potential of the kundalini is perceived to reside at the base of the central channel in the pelvis.

On either side of the sushumna or central channel are two important currents in which Prana flows called the ida and pingala or, respectively, the lunar and solar channels. These two lateral channels are representative of the polarized passive and active forces or energies, similar to the concepts of Yin and Yang. The lunar and solar channels are connected to the nostrils and the mechanism of breathing, the breath being the physical source for nourishing and expressing the Prana. The two channels are said to approximate or communicate with each other along the sushumna, resulting in the generation of a chakra, literally meaning a wheel.

Classically there are seven main chakras located within the sushumna. Each chakra is the focal point of primal forces, including subtle aspects of mind, karmic restrictions, extremely refined Prana, and the pure spirit. Classical symbols are used in Tantra to describe these forces found within the chakras. The most important symbols associated with the individual chakras are elements, petals, geometric design, color, and sound, which together denote a chakra's vibrational potency and position. In addition, each chakra is connected to a particular deity that metaphorically describes its psychodynamic nature.

In the mystical Tantric path the adept tries to potentize and then merge the two lateral channels, followed by withdrawing their combined force into the sushumna. This is achieved through the use of special breathing techniques, visualizations, ritual, intent and other means.

Buddhist Tantra

In Asia, there are many differing forms of Tantra, although most are based upon and in agreement with the Hindu approach to Tantra. Especially noteworthy are the Buddhist schools of Tantra. In particular, the Vajrayana sect of Tibetan Buddhism is noted for its rich commentary on the sushumna and chakras, as well as on all aspects of incarnation and karma.

Generally, Buddhist teachings on the inner dimension utilize a different set of symbolic images to explain the contents and nature of the sushumna and chakras than does Hinduism. In the Tibetan tradition the location and number of chakras are also different from the Hindu teachings. Within the Hindu tradition, most schools describe the sushumna as occupying the space that over-laps the innermost core of the spine and brain. The Buddhists, on the other hand, believe the sushumna is superimposed upon the physical space anterior to the spinal column, near the center of the body's trunk and head. Furthermore, while there are seven principal chakras mentioned in the Hindu tantric teachings, only five main centers (and sometimes a sixth, the Crown center) are spoken of in the Buddhist approach.

Regarding this variation between the Hindu and Buddhist teachings on the chakras, Lama Anagarika Govinda, in his book *Foundations of Tibetan Mysticism*, comments:

> "The main difference between the two systems lies in the different treatment of the same fundamental facts. Just as travelers of different temperaments or of different interests and mental attitudes would describe the same landscape in quite different ways, without contradicting thereby each other or the given facts, in the same way the Buddhist and Hindu followers of Tantra invest the same landscapes of the human mind with different experiences."

In Lama Govinda's view, the Hindu system emphasizes the correspondences between each chakra and its primary element, symbols and cosmic forces. Furthermore, these objective contents are thought to be permanently fixed. In comparison, the Buddhist system is less concerned with the static and objective aspects of the chakras; rather the focus is on what flows through them and their dynamic functions. Therefore in the Buddhist tradition sounds, colors or other symbols are not considered permanent features of a chakra. It is believed that the contents of the chakras along the sushumna may interact, mutually penetrate and combine with each other under certain conditions, such as by intention during spiritual training or in a spontaneous awakening.

Ayurveda

The third science, Ayurveda, literally means the knowledge of life. Ayurveda is a holistic medical art that primarily strives to address the well being of mind and body. Grounded in the Samkhya philosophy, Ayurveda utilizes a tri-dosha doctrine to explain how ill health and disease manifest.

According to Ayurveda's tri-dosha theory, the five elements manifest within the body as three quintessential substances: essence, Prana and a subtle fire. Prana is the life force that vitalizes, connects and harmonizes the physical, mental and causal spheres. Essence is the biological force and ground matrix of the physical body. The subtle fire is a transformative force that allows the body's various substances to undergo change. The subtle fire is often imagined as the catalyst in the digestive, metabolic, and nervous system processes. These three quintessential substances create the basis for all the other bodily substances and tissues. Prana and essence are largely equivalent to the Chinese concepts of Qi and essence.

Prana, subtle fire, and essence are too subtle to satisfy all of the body's demands, so they metamorphose into doshas, literally meaning fault. The three doshas - vata, pitta and kapha - are grosser manifestations of Prana, subtle fire, and essence. In healthy balance the doshas aid in the maintenance and integration of all the mind and body's functions, while an imbalance of one or more doshas generates disturbance and disorder.

The doctrine of the doshas is fundamental to Ayurveda's explanation of how each human being develops a unique constitution or temperament. At birth, each individual will have a tendency towards a deficiency or excess of one or more doshas. Rare is the person with all their doshas balanced. This acquired tendency will determine to a large extent the personality, desired lifestyle, physical shape, health and well being of that individual.

During life, balanced doshas may become imbalanced and imbalanced doshas aggravated through the inappropriate use of foods, thoughts and activities, as well as injuries and environmental illnesses. Since no two people will have the exact same constitutional pattern or illness, what is appropriate for each person will be different.

Furthermore, Ayurveda states that the three doshas have particular qualities and tendencies that exist both within and outside of people. Essentially, vata is considered dry, cold, light, rough and unstable; pitta is oily, hot, light, intense and mobile; kapha is oily, cold, heavy, smooth and stable. When taken into the body, any substance will increase a dosha's presence and activity, if the substance has similar attributes to that dosha. For example, ice cream, a substance with kapha qualities, will naturally increase the presence of mucus, cool the body and engender heaviness by encouraging body fat. If a person already had too much kapha in their constitution or is suffering from a kapha-like illness, then avoiding ice cream would be best. Substances are not, however, limited to just one dosha; they may contain two or all three.

Ayurveda aspires to help individuals live their life in the fullest way possible according to their constitution. Often this requires a long term strategy in treatment and prevention. Nevertheless, life is often full of crises and acute illnesses. Ayurveda does not neglect the immediate necessities. It has developed excellent strategies and treatment of the myriad of health concerns, all of which are based upon the concept of the doshas.

For both constitutional and acute care, Ayurveda incorporates various modalities, such as the use of plant, mineral and animal medicines; the use of prayer and mantras; dietary counsel; massage; bone-setting and surgery; bloodletting; cauterization; plus various adjunctive techniques.

Today there is intense interest in Ayurvedic medicine throughout the world. Perhaps this is due to Ayurveda's inherent simplicity, effectiveness, and reliance on a theory that is based on unchanging laws of nature. In my experience, the tri-dosha concept is easily and naturally understood by people everywhere; it is not limited to the Indian culture. This is, I believe, because the doshas are based upon an inherent biological pattern that is part and parcel of our physical development.

Alchemy. (*Chinese: wei-nei dan*) In the Chinese version, alchemy is an extension of Taoism which seeks immortality and spiritual enrichment through manipulating matter and time.

Anima-Animus. According to Jungian psychology, anima is the inner feminine side of a man, while animus is the inner masculine side of a woman. They can be experienced as either an archetypal image (see below) or a personal complex, an emotionally charged group of thoughts and memories.

Archetype. A primordial structural pattern of the mind, especially within the infraconscious aspect (*see below*). The image of a "Gaia, the Earth Mother" or "anima-animus" (*see above*) are examples of archetypes.

Aura. An energetic protective barrier that is projected outside the skin's surface. The aura has various layers; however, the most important layer is the etheric aura. This layer protects the body and mind.

Bardo. (Tibetan) Literally, an "in-between state." Any transitory stage of existence or reality. Most often associated with death, rebirth, and the intermediary realm between.

Blastocyst. The stage of the embryo's development when it is largely spherical in shape (with a fluid filled cavity) and composed of undifferentiated cells.

Chakra. (Sanskrit) Literally, a "wheel." Chakras are sites where subtle aspects of consciousness gather along the Sushumna (*see above*).

Derm. Refers to the embryo's primary tissue layers, called the endo, ecto and meso derm that manifest with gastrulation (*see below*). They are the origin of the physical body's tissues, organs and systems.

Doshas. (Sanskrit) Literally, "a fault." The Doshas of Ayurveda are grosser forms of Prana, Subtle Fire, and Essence (*see below*) which appear in the body as condensations of the Five Elements (*see below*). There are three Doshas: Vata, Pitta and Kapha.

Energy vortex. A psychic complex of strong energetic potency that is lodged within the body's tissues. These vortices usually contain latent feelings and memories which are the result of traumas and unintegrated experiences.

Essence. (*Chinese: jing / Sanskrit: ojas*) A concept that is inherent in both Chinese Medicine and Ayurveda. Essence refers to the body's biological matrix and reproductive capacity. Its visible form is the sperm and egg. Throughout life, "essence" controls the basal vitality and physical cohesion of the tissues.

Fascia. A form of connective tissue that lines most bodily structures, like the muscles, tendons, bones, brain and organs.

Fields of Influence. (*Chinese: dan tian*) In Taoism, there are three energetic sites within the body where internal substances (Essence, Qi, and Spirit) are gathered and transformed. They correspond to the Brow, Heart and Vitality centers of the psychoenergetic core.

Five Elements. (*Chinese: wu xing / Sanskrit: pancha mahabhuta*) The Chinese and Indian traditions use a Five Element model to explain the workings of nature. They are archetypal images through which to express ideas. Although both traditions identify five basic elements, they are, however, dissimilar in most ways. Even the elements they identify are different. The Chinese use the elements metal, wood, earth, water and fire, while the Indians use ether, air, fire, water and earth in their model.

Gastrulation. A stage of the embryo's development when the derm cells start to differentiate and pattern themselves.

Infraconscious. That which is below the conscious mind's threshold of awareness. The infraconscious is composed of two parts: the personal and transpersonal aspects (*see below*). The infraconscious has been referred to as the "unconscious" mind.

Karma. (Sanskrit) Literally, "action." Put simply, karma refers to a chain of cause and effect. In human beings, karma is traceable to the patterns of thought and action.

Knots. (*Sanskrit: granthi*) In Tantra, this term refers to the three psychoenergetic centers in which karmic restrictions tend to be more pronounced. They are the Brow, Heart and Vitality centers.

Kundalini Shakti. (Sanskrit) Literally, the "serpent power." A latent primordial potential that lies at the bottom of the Sushumna (*see below*). The kundalini represents the soul's enclosure in form, time and space.

Mandala. (Sanskrit) Literally, a "circle or arch." In both Hindu and Buddhist Tantra (*see below*) mandalas are used as symbolic representations of cosmic and divine forces. In psychology, such a symbol represents a striving for unity in the self.

Meridians. (*Chinese: jing*) The subtle channels through which Qi or energy flows. The practice of acupuncture and acupressure are based upon the meridian concept.

Nadi. (Sanskrit) The subtle channels through which Prana moves, similar to the idea of the meridians (*see above*).

Personal Infraconscious. An intermediary stage between the conscious mind and the transpersonal infraconscious (*see below*). Its primarily function is to store thoughts not yet ripe for consciousness, lost or repressed memories, or subliminal perceptions that contain impressions of past events. Often referred to as the "personal unconscious" by Jungian analysts.

Potentize. To charge and vibrationally uplift energy or matter from one state to another.

Prana. (Sanskrit) Literally, the "breath of life." The human life force or energy. Virtually identical to the Chinese concept of Qi (*see below*).

Qi. (Chinese) Literally, "energy or breath." Denotes the inherent life force or energy that animates the body. Qi is differentiated according to its various functions and/or locations. For example, organ Qi, defensive Qi, meridian Qi, and so on.

Quaternity. An emblem for the mind's way to orient itself based on a fourfold pattern.

Rebirth. When consciousness or spirit is born into a new body, in its journey through many lives.

Rishi. (Sanskrit) A seer of truth; a realized person or saint.

Samadhi. (Sanskrit) A supraconscious state in which divine union or at-oneness is realized.

Shaman. An indigenous medicine man and/or a priest. Often used in reference to those who use the forces of nature and the supranatural to evoke healing.

Somatic. Relating to the physical body as distinct from the mind, energy and spirit.

Subtle. A refined form of energy, not obvious to the usual physical senses; an apprehension requiring a shift of awareness to perceive it.

Subtle Fire. (*Sanskrit: tejas*) The transformative potential that allows influences and substances to pass from one plane of existence to another.

Supraconscious. A state of cosmic consciousness that is above or beyond the individual mind. A mystical realm of pure spirit.

Sushumna. (Sanskrit) Literally, the "central conduit." The immaterial divine core within human beings. It contains seven chakras or psychic centers that house spirit and mind, and serves to differentiate consciousness.

Synchronicity. Meaningful personal or global events that coincide within the same time period, suggesting purposeful designed intent.

Syntonic. A profound feeling of harmony with life, including one's immediate environment.

Tantra. (Sanskrit) Literally, a "continuum or context." Tantra teaches that the universe is composed of two aspects: a feminine (Shakti) primal force and a masculine (Shiva) state of pure awareness. The followers of Tantra try to reconcile these two aspects within themselves.

Tao. (Chinese) Literally, the "way." In Chinese philosophy, the Tao denotes the source of creation. The Tao has a passive aspect, the Void (*see below*), which is an unmanifest creative potential that gives rise to its active aspect, the Great Ultimate, a manifest generative force.

Temperament. The human constitution based upon biological and behavioral characteristics.

Transpersonal Infraconscious. An aspect of consciousness that is a repository of humanity's psychological evolution and a wellspring for human creativity. This level of the infraconscious (*see above*) is often expressed in the form of primordial, mythological and spiritual images. Often referred to as the "collective or transpersonal unconscious" by Jungian analysts.

Vibrational Frequencies. The subtle rates of oscillation or movement which occur in all phenomena, from the subatomic level to sound and light.

Visualization. A form of guided imagery that can be used to expand awareness and facilitate healing.

Void. (*Chinese: wu*) The unmanifest creative capacity and passive aspect of the Tao (*see above*). Considered to be beyond the material universe, yet the cause of it.

Yang. (Chinese) Literally, the "light." The positive principle from nature's primal duality.

Yantra. (Sanskrit) Literally, "support or instrument." A sacred geometric design or diagram used in India as a symbol for spiritual purposes.

Yin. (Chinese) Literally, the "dark." The negative principle from nature's primal duality.

Yoga. (Sanskrit) Literally, "to bind together." Usually Yoga refers to the ancient Hindu sciences of spirituality. Any path of knowledge that leads to union with God can be called Yoga.

Acupuncture: A Chinese healing art that utilizes needles, finger pressure (acupressure) and mild cauterization (moxibustion) to stimulate the Qi flow within a network of subtle meridians under the skin.

Suggested reading: *The Layman's Guide to Acupuncture* by Yoshio Manaka and Ian Urquhart (Weatherhill, 1984).

Ayurveda: An enduring three thousand year old Indian science of healing whose core teachings are recorded in a number of revered classics, the principal text being the Caraka Samhita (circa 800 B.C.). Ayurveda offers a holistic approach to understanding, recognizing and treating disease, and in leading a balanced vital lifestyle according to each person's unique constitution. The main therapies are diet, botanical and mineral medicines, massage, and purification therapy.

Suggested reading: *Ayurveda: A Holistic Approach to Health and Longevity* by Judith Morrison (Fireside Book, 1995).

Chinese Medicine: A pragmatic blend of various ancient Chinese healing practices that incorporate an understanding of mankind's connection to nature and to nature's source, the Tao. These ideas are aptly expounded in the Yellow Emperor's Inner Classic (circa 200 B.C.). Primarily, Chinese medicine consists of two branches: internal medicine, which uses natural medicines, mostly of plant, animal, and mineral sources and dietary advice; and, external medicine, that includes massage, joint manipulation, acupuncture and moxibustion.

Suggested reading: *Between Heaven and Earth: A Guide to Chinese Medicine* by Harriet Beinfield and Efrem Korngold (Ballantine Books, 1991).

For a comparison and summary of these two Asian systems of medicine, please read: *Tao & Dharma: Chinese Medicine and Ayurveda* by Arnie Lade and Robert Svoboda (Lotus Press, 1995).

Cardio-energetics: An emerging field that uses findings from medical disciplines (such as cardiology, neurology, psychology and psychoneuroimmunology) and the basic principles of quantum physics to explore the role of the heart in conveying and communicating energy and subtle information.

Suggested reading: *The Heart's Code* by Paul Pearsall (Broadway Books, 1997)

Craniosacral Manipulation: In this healing art, special manipulative techniques are used to treat disorders that arise from or impact upon the cranial system. Craniosacral manipulation was developed by osteopaths and uses gentle hands-on procedures to correct functional restrictions within the cranium, spine, and throughout the fascial system.

Suggested reading: *Craniosacral Therapy* by John Upledger and Jon Vredevoogd (Eastland Press, 1983).

Feldenkrais Method: Movements subtle and gross, are the major expression of the human brain and mind. Most human movement is learned and colored by the emotional atmosphere in which it was acquired, rather then inherited. The Feldenkrais method is a way to enlarge the repertoire and revive patterns of movement for pain relief, improved physical and artistic performance, or grace and pleasure in daily life.

Suggested reading: *Awareness Heals: The Feldenkrais Method for Dynamic Health* by Steven Shafarman (Addison-Wesley Publishing Co., Inc., 1997)

Jin Shin Do: A unique synthesis of acupressure, western psychology, and Taoist philosophy based upon the work of Iona Teeguarden. This is a gentle mind-body approach for working with Qi.

Suggested reading: *The Joy of Feeling - Bodymind Acupressure* by Iona Teeguarden (Japan Publications, 1987).

Jungian Psychology: A form of psychological analysis that aims to reconnect the patient to his or her inner Self, the center of both wholeness and individuality. In therapy, archetypes or instinctive patterns of both the conscious and infraconscious mind, as revealed in one's dream life, are used to address specific problems and to understand the Self.

Suggested reading: *Boundaries of the Soul* by June Singer (Doubleday, 1972).

Music Therapy: The power of healing through sound and music is as old as civilization itself. This is a fascinating field that is only now becoming accepted and seriously researched.

Suggested reading: *Sounding the Inner Landscape* by Kay Gardner (Caduceus Publications, 1990).

Polarity Therapy: In this eclectic discipline, eastern Ayurvedic philosophy has been blended with western science and natural healing arts. Polarity is based on the theory of subtle life energy and its manifestations that was developed by Randolf Stone in the early 1950's. Manual therapy is used to balance energy and forms the basis of treatment. Nutrition, exercise and attitudinal training are used as adjunctive aides.

Suggested reading: *The Polarity Process* by Franklyn Stills (Element Books, 1989).

Qi Gong: A popular Chinese practice that utilizes breathing and gentle, rhythmic movement to improve vitality and restore health.

Suggested reading: *Living Qigong* by John Alton (Shambhala Publications, 1997).

Tai Ji Quan: Though considered a Chinese martial art, Tai Ji Quan is closely aligned with Taoist philosophy and is taught as a graceful set of movements that enhances mental and physical well being. There are numerous traditions, each emphasizing different styles of movement, although mastering the Qi is at the heart of this practice.

Suggested reading: *Embracing Tiger Return to Mountain: The Essence of Tai Ji* by Al Huang (Celestial Arts Press, 1987).

Taoist Inner Alchemy: A divergent group of practices are embraced under Taoist Inner Alchemy, including meditation and visualization techniques, breathing and movement exercises, sexual disciplines and longevity practices. All methods aim to promote self-healing and to align the individual with the Tao, the source of all things.

Suggested reading: *Awakening Healing Energy Through the Tao* by Mantak Chia (Aurora Press, 1983).

Visceral Manipulation: Disorders within the organs have both local and systemic implications within the body. Visceral manipulation uses special techniques to re-establish order. This science and art was developed, mainly, through the work of the French osteopath, Dr. J.P. Barral.

Suggested reading: *Visceral Manipulation* by Jean-Pierre Barral and Pierre Mercier (Eastland Press, 1988).

Yoga: There are many forms of Indian Yoga which have been exported throughout the world. Hatha Yoga, involving gentle stretching exercises, breathing, and awareness, is by far the most common form of Yoga practiced in the West.

Suggested reading: *Yoga for a Better Life* by David Schonfeld (Quest Publications, 1980).

Somatoenergetics is a healing art based upon the principles outlined in this book. "Somato" refers to our embodied physical forms, "energetics" to the study of energy and its transformations, and together they denote the study of the embodied life force or energy within us. Somatoenergetics offers an integral approach to health, the understanding of illness and restoration of well being, as well as the relationship between mind and body. In its practice, Somatoenergetics incorporates energetic theory, assessment skills, hands-on healing techniques, diet, and natural therapeutics. These practices are adapted from both ancient and modern sources, and integrated with the theory of energy according to the experience of its developer, Arnie Lade. Somatoenergetics is an evolving, eclectic discipline, one that promotes an attitude of infinite learning and loving kindness.

For more information about workshops and professional training programs, please write to:

Somatoenergetics
PO Box 8621
Victoria, BC
V8W 3S2
Canada
or visit the author's website:
www. energetichealing.com

Alpin, J. Van; *Oriental Medicine;* Shambhala
Publications, 1995; Boston, U.S.A.

Avalon, A.; *The Serpent Power;* Dover Publications,
1919; New York, U.S.A.

Barral, J.P. and Mercier, P.; *Visceral Manipulation;*
Eastland Press, 1988; Seattle, U.S.A.

Beinfield, H. & Korngold, E.; *Between Heaven and Earth
- A Guide to Chinese Medicine;* Ballantine Books, 1991;
New York, U.S.A.

Beaulieu, J.; *Music and Sound in the Healing Arts;*
Station Hill Press, 1987; Barrytown, U.S.A.

Bendit, L. & Bendit, P.; *The Etheric Body of Man;*
Theosophical Publishing House, 1957; Wheaton, U.S.A.

Bott, V.; *Anthroposophical Medicine;* Rudolf Steiner
Press, 1978; London, U.K.

Breaux, C.; *Journey Into Consciousness - The Chakras,
Tantra and Jungian Psychology;* Nicholas-Hays, Inc.,
1989; York Beach, U.S.A.

Cabrera, J.; *The Message of the Engraved Stones of Ica;*
J.C.D. Press, 1988; Ica, Peru.

Campbell, J.; *The Inner Reaches of Outer Space -
Metaphor as Myth and As Religion;* Harper & Row,
Inc.,1986: New York, U.S.A.

Campbell, J.; *The Mythic Image;* Princeton University
Press, 1974; Princeton, U.S.A.

Carlson, J.B.; *America's Ancient Skywatchers;* Journal
of the National Geographic Society; March, 1990;
Washington, U.S.A.

Chang, G.; *Tibetan Yoga;* Citadel Press, 1993; Newark,
U.S.A.

Chinese Academy of Sciences; *Ancient China's Technology and Science;* Foreign Language Press, 1983; Beijing, China.

Chia, M.; *Awaken Healing Energy Through The Tao;* Aurora Press, 1983; New York, U.S.A.

Cohen, D.; *An Introduction to Craniosacral Therapy;* North Atlantic Books, 1995; Berkeley, U.S.A.

Cooper, J.C.; Taoism: *The Way of the Mystic;* Mandala 1972; London, U.K.

Coward, H.; *Jung and Eastern Thought;* State University of New York Press, 1985; Albany, U.S.A.

Eliade, M.; *Yoga - Immortality and Freedom;* Princeton University Press, 1969; Princeton, U.S.A.

Feng G.F. & English, J.; *Lao Tsu - Tao Te Ching;* Random House, 1972; New York, U.S.A

Fregtman, C.D.; *Holomusica;* Editorial Kairos, 1988; Barcelona, Spain.

Freemantle, F. & Trungpa, C.; *The Tibetan Book of the Dead;* Shambhala Publications, 1987; Boston, U.S.A.

Gardner, K.; *Sounding the Inner Landscape: Music and Medicine;* Caduceus Publications, 1990; Stonington, U.S.A.

Groff, S. & Bennett, H.Z.; *The Holotropic Mind;* Harper-Collins, 1990, New York, U.S.A.

Jaggi, O.P.; *History of Science, Technology and Medicine in India: Volume 2 - Ayurveda: Indian System of Medicine, Volume 5 - Yogic and Tantric Medicine, Volume 8 - Medicine in Medieval India;* Atma Ram & Sons, 1981; Delhi, India.

Jenning, H.; Cymatics: *The Structure and Dynamics of Waves and Vibrations,* Volume 1 & 2; Basilius Press, 1967; Basil, Switzerland.

Johari, H.; Chakras: *Energy Centers of Transformation;* Destiny Books, 1983; Rochester, U.S.A.

Jung, C.G.; *Man and His Symbols;* Anchor Books, Doubleday, 1964; New York, U.S.A.

Jung, C.G.; *Memories, Dreams, Reflections;* Vintage Books, 1989; New York, U.S.A

Kakar, S.; *Shamans, Mystics and Doctors;* University of Chicago Press, 1982; Chicago, U.S.A.

Khanna, M.; *Yantra: The Tantric Symbol of Cosmic Unity;* Thames and Hudson, 1979; New York, U.S.A.

Lade, A.; *Acupuncture Points: Images & Functions;* Eastland Press, 1989; Seattle, U.S.A.

Lade, A. and Svoboda, R.; *Tao & Dharma: Chinese Medicine and Ayurveda;* Lotus Press, 1995;

Twin Lakes, U.S.A.

Larsen, W.; *Human Embryology;* Churchill Livingstone, 1993; New York, U.S.A.

Lati, R. & Hopkins, J.; *Death, Intermediate State and Rebirth in Tibetan Buddhism;* Snow Lion, 1979; Ithaca, U.S.A.

Leadbeater, C.W.; *The Chakras;* The Theosophical Publishing House, 1927; Wheaton, U.S.A.

Levine, S.; *Who Dies? An Investigation into Conscious Living and Conscious Dying;* Anchor Books, Doubleday, 1982; New York, U.S.A.

Liu, Y.C.; *The Essential Book of Traditional Chinese Medicine; Volume 1 - Theory; Volume 2 - Clinical Practice;* Columbia University Press, 1988; New York, U.S.A.

Lodo, L.; *Bardo Teachings: The Way of Death and Rebirth;* Snow Lion, 1987; Ithaca, U.S.A.

Luk, C.; *Taoist Yoga;* Samuel Weiser, Inc, 1970; York Beach, U.S.A.

Lyons, A.S. & Petrucelli, R.J.; *Medicine: An Illustrated History;* Abrams, 1987: New York, U.S.A.

Magoun, H.I.; *Osteopathy in the Cranial Field;* The Sutherland Cranial Teaching foundation, 1966; Belen, U.S.A.

Matsumoto, K. & Birch, S.; *Hara Diagnosis: Reflections on the Sea;* Paradigm Publications, 1988; Brookline, U.S.A.

Mees, L.F.C.: *Secrets of the Skeleton;* Anthroposophical Press, 1984; Spring Valley, U.S.A.

Men, H.; *Secrets of Mayan Science/Religion;* Bear & Company, 1989; Santa Fe, U.S.A.

Morrison, J.H.; *The Book of Ayurveda;* Fireside Book, 1995; New York, U.S.A.

Mookerjee, A.; *Kundalini - the Arousal of the Inner Energy;* Destiny Books, 1982; Rochester, U.S.A.

Mookerjee, A. & Khanna, M.; *The Tantric Way;* Thames and Hudson, 1977; London, U.K.

Motoyama, H.; *Theories of the Chakras: Bridge to Higher Consciousness;* The Theosophical Publishing House; Wheaton, U.S.A.

Motoyama, H. & Brown, R.; *Science and Evolution of Consciousness - Chakras, Ki and Psi;* Autumn Press, 1978; Brookline, U.S.A.

O'Flaherty, W.D.; *The Rig Veda;* Penguin Books, 1981; London, U.K.

Sheldon, W.H.; *The Varieties of Temperament;* Harper & Brothers Publishers, 1942; New York, U.S.A.

Sills, F.; *The Polarity Process;* Element Books, 1989; Longmead, U.K.

Sogyal Rimpoche; *The Tibetan Book of Living and Dying;* Harper-Collins Publishers, 1992; New York, U.S.A.

Steiner, R.; *At The Gates of Spiritual Science;* Rudolf Steiner Press, 1970; London, U.K.

Steiner, R.; *Spiritual Science and Medicine;* Rudolf Steiner Press, 1948; London, U.K.

Stone, R.; *Polarity Therapy - New Energy Concept of the Healing Arts: Book 2 - The Wireless Anatomy of Man,* 1953; Book 3 - *Polarity Therapy,* 1954; Pannetier Publishing; Orange County, U.S.A.

Sutherland, W.G.;*Teachings in the Science of Osteopathy;* Rudra Press & Sutherland Cranial Teaching Foundation, Inc., 1990; Fort Worth, U.S.A.

Tobyn, G.; *Culpeper's Medicine: A Practice of Western Holistic Medicine;* Element Books, 1997; Rockport, U.S.A.

Udupa, K.N. & Singh, R.N. (editors); *Science and Philosophy of Indian Medicine;* Shree Baidyanath Ayurved Bhawan Ltd, 1978; Nagpur, India.

Unschuld, P.U.; *Medicine in China, A History of Ideas;* University of California Press, 1985; Berkeley, U.S.A.

Upledger, J.E. & Vredevoogd, J.D.; *Craniosacral Therapy;* Eastland Press, 1983; Seattle, U.S.A.

Upledger, J.E.; *A Brain Is Born;* North Atlantic Press & UI Enterprises, 1996; Berkeley, U.S.A.

Von Franz, M.L.; *Psyche and Matter;* Shambhala Press, 1992; Boston, U.S.A.

Vieth, I.; *The Yellow Emperor's Classic of Internal Medicine;* University of California Press, 1949; Berkeley, U.S.A.

Wolpert, L.; *The Triumph of the Embryo;* Oxford University Press, 1991; New York, U.S.A.

Ywahoo, D.; *Voices of Our Ancestors:* Shambhala Press, 1987; Boston, U.S.A.

Sources of Illustrations

8-2 Reprinted from *Visceral Manipulation* by Jean-Pierre Barral and Pierre Mercier with permission of Eastland Press, PO Box 12689, Seattle, WA 98111. Copyright 1988. All rights reserved.

8-5 Reprinted from *Craniosacral Therapy* by John Upledger and Jon Vredevoogd with permission of Eastland Press, PO Box 12689, Seattle, WA 98111. Copyright 1983. All rights reserved.

8-6 Reprinted from *The Thorax* by Jean-Pierre Barral with permission of Eastland Press, PO Box 12689, Seattle, WA 98111. Copyright 1991. All rights reserved.

9-1 & 9-3 Reprinted from *Chinese Massage Therapy* by Anhui Medical School, Vancouver, BC: Hartley and Marks, 1987. All rights reserved.

SOURCE OF QUOTES

Page 9: Joseph Campbell: *The Power of Myth* (New York, NY: Doubleday, 1988) Material used by permission.

Pages 14-15: Joseph Campbell: *The Inner Reaches of Outer Space* (New York, NY: Harper & Row, 1986) Material used by permission.

Pages 47 & 236: Lama Anagarika Govinda: *Foundations of Tibetan Mysticism* (York Beach, ME: Samuel Weiser, 1969) Material used by permission.

Page 212: C.G. Jung: *Memories, Dreams, Reflections* (New York, NY: Random House, 1989) Material used by permission.

LIST OF ILLUSTRATIONS

INDEX

ABOUT THE AUTHOR

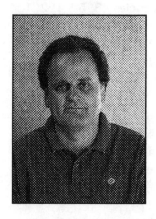

Arnie Lade is an acupuncturist and specialist in energetic healing. He originally trained in massage, botanical medicine, and manipulative therapies, before studying acupuncture in China. Arnie resides with his family in Victoria, Canada, lecturing and traveling widely. He is the author of *Acupuncture Points: Images & Functions*, and co-author of *Chinese Exercise and Massage*, and *Tao & Dharma: Chinese Medicine and Ayurveda*.

Herbs and other natural health products and information are often available at natural food stores or metaphysical bookstores. If you cannot find what you need locally, you can contact one of the follwing sources of supply.

Sources of Supply:

The following companies have an extensive selection of useful products and a long track-record of fulfillment. They have natural body care, aromatherapy, flower essences, crystals and tumbled stones, homeopathy, herbal products, vitamins and supplements, videos, books, audio tapes, candles, incense and bulk herbs, teas, massage tools and products and numerous alternative health items across a wide range of categories.

WHOLESALE:

Wholesale suppliers sell to stores and practitioners, not to individual consumers buying for their own personal use. Individual consumers should contact the RETAIL supplier listed below. Wholesale accounts should contact with business name, resale number or practitioner license in order to obtain a wholesale catalog and set up an account.

Lotus Light Enterprises, Inc.

P O Box 1008 EH
Silver Lake, WI 53170 USA
414 889 8501 (phone)
414 889 8591 (fax)
800 548 3824 (toll free order line)

RETAIL:

Retail suppliers provide products by mail order direct to consumers for their personal use. Stores or practitioners should contact the wholesale supplier listed above.

Internatural

33719 116th Street EH
Twin Lakes, WI 53181 USA
800 643 4221 (toll free order line)
414 889 8581 office phone
WEB SITE: www.internatural.com

Web site includes an extensive annotated catalog of more than 7000 products that can be ordered "on line" for your convenience 24 hours a day, 7 days a week.

Tao and Dharma
Chinese Medicine and Ayurveda
by Robert Svoboda and Arnie Lade
Foreward by Michael Tierra, O.M.D.

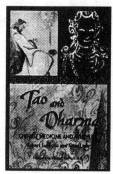

"Taoism is a highly spiritual and mystical way of trandscending the human realm. Chinese medicine, whose roots embrace the Tao, provides a fundamental understanding of the reality of individual life. Ayurveda is the knowledge of life, an ancient Vedic art of balancing individual life in harmony with nature. Chinese medicine and Ayurveda are concurrent and inherent systems of healing every individual as he or she is. Together, Robert Svoboda and Arnie Lade have done remarkable work in order to bring forth the prospect of integral healing through the ancient Vedic and Oriental systems of medicine." Dr. Vasant Lad, author of Ayurveda: Science of Self Healing

"Traditional Chinese and Ayurvedic medicine constitute the two major legacies for health and healing from the ancient world....the Taoist Yin-Yang philosophy and the three Doshas of Ayurveda...were used according to their respective cultural contexts to determine the most balanced and appropriate diet, herbs, exercise and lifestyle according to inherited constitution, life work and climate....In these times of maximum fragmentation, it is truly a miracle that the perennial truths and the healing capacities of these great ancient philosophies can arise....

"To this purpose, this valuable work should serve as an important contribution."
Michael Tierra, O.M.D., author of Planetary Herbology, Chinese Traditional Herbal Medicine, and The Way of Herbs

This book's interesting and valuable comparison provides a pioneering effort in examining side by side two great systems of medicine, studying closely the historical, theoretical and practical relationships. In so doing, it offers these ancient paradigms for a synergistic, inclusive approach into the practice of modern healing.

To order your copy send $12.95 plus $3.00 shipping/handling ($1.50 for each additional copy) to Lotus Press, P O Box 325, Twin Lakes, WI 53181 USA 800 824 6396 email: lotuspress@lotuspress.com website: www.lotuspress.com

Wisconsin residents add appropriate sales tax for your county. Wholesale inquiries welcome. Visa, Mastercard, American Express and Discover accepted.

Lotus Press is the publisher of a wide range of books in the field of alternative health, including ayurveda, chinese medicine, herbology, aromatherapy, and energetic healing modalities. Request our free book catalog.

ISBN 0-914955-21-7   155 pp.   trade paper $12.95

Lotus Press, P.O. Box 325 EH, Twin Lakes, WI 53181 • 800-824-6396 (order line)
414-889-8561 (office phone) •414-889-8591 (fax line)
e-mail: lotuspress@lotuspress.com web site: www.lotuspress.com